- Clinical Nutrition

DIET THERAPY FOR DIGESTIVE DISEASES

Practical Guide for Nutritionists

FIRST EDITION

Dr. Amin Gasmi

© **Copyright 2020 by Dr. Amin Gasmi - All rights reserved.**

The contents of this book may not be reproduced, duplicated or transmitted without direct written permission from the author.

Under no circumstances will any legal responsibility or blame be held against the publisher for any reparation, damages, or monetary loss due to the information herein, either directly or indirectly.

Legal Notice:

This book is copyright protected. This is only for personal use. You cannot amend, distribute, sell, use, quote or paraphrase any part or the content within this book without the consent of the author.

Disclaimer Notice:

Please note the information contained within this document is for educational and entertainment purposes only. Every attempt has been made to provide accurate, up to date and reliable complete information. No warranties of any kind are expressed or implied. Readers acknowledge that the author is not engaging in the rendering of legal, financial, medical or professional advice. The content of this book has been derived from various sources. Please consult a licensed professional before attempting any techniques outlined in this book.

By reading this document, the reader agrees that under no circumstances is the author responsible for any losses, direct or indirect, which are incurred as a result of the use of information contained within this document, including, but not limited to, —errors, omissions, or inaccuracies.

DEDICATION

To the ultimate power of the universe, the power of love. For me, more than all: dad, mom, my wife, Alain, Cherif and Salva.

ACKNOWLEDGEMENT

I thank all those who throughout my life have contributed to my training and make me what I have become today: God, my family, my teachers, my colleagues, my friends, my students, my patients, my athletes, and everyone I have met on my way. I am also indebted to a large number of books and scientific articles, and I cannot thank their authors enough for their sharing and generosity.

TABLE OF CONTENTS

Dedication iii

Acknowledgement iv

1.0 Clinical Nutrition for Diseases of the Esophagus, Stomach, and Duodenum 1

    1.1   Principles of Clinical Nutrition 2

    1.2   Basics of Clinical Nutrition for Diseases of the Esophagus, Stomach, and Duodenum 5

2.0 Clinical Nutrition for Diseases of the Liver and Biliary Tract 28

    2.1   General Recommendations 29

    2.2   Acute Cholecystitis, Exacerbation of Chronic Cholecystitis 32

    2.3   Chronic Cholecystitis without Exacerbation 33

    2.4   Gallstone Disease 34

    2.5   Acute Hepatitis 36

    2.6   Chronic Hepatitis 37

    2.7   Cirrhosis 39

    2.8   Hepatic Encephalopathy 40

    2.9   Ascites 42

    2.10   Alcoholic Liver Disease 43

    2.11   Wilson – Konovalov's Disease. 45

3.0 Clinical Nutrition for Diseases of the Pancreas 46

- 3.1 Acute Pancreatitis and Exacerbation of Chronic Pancreatitis 47
- 3.2 Remission Phase of Acute and Chronic Pancreatitis 51
- 3.3 Chronic Pancreatitis with Incretory Insufficiency 53
- 3.4 Sample Menus 55

4.0 Clinical Nutrition for Bowel Diseases 57

- 4.1 Basics of Clinical Nutrition for Intestinal Disorders 58
- 4.2 Diarrhea Syndrome 61
- 4.3 Intestinal Dyspepsia 63
- 4.4 Diseases of the Intestine with Diarrhea 67
- 4.5 Constipation Syndrome 69
- 4.6 Excessive Gas Formation in the Intestine 74
- 4.7 Diverticular Bowel Disease 74
- 4.8 Fermentopathies (enzyme deficiency enteropathies) 76

5.0 Clinical Nutrition After Operations On The Digestive Organs ... 99

- 5.1 After Surgery on the Esophagus 101
- 5.2 After Surgery on the Stomach and Duodenum 107
- 5.3 Post-Gastroresection Syndromes 108
- 5.4 After Bowel Surgery 114
- 5.5 After Surgery on the Liver 120
- 5.6 After Surgery on the Biliary Tract 121
- 5.7 After Pancreatic Surgery 124

6.0 Technical Diet Models for Digestive Diseases..........................127

    6.1   Diet N°1 127

    6.2   Diet N°2 144

    6.3   Diet N°3 148

    6.4   Diet N°4 155

    6.5   Diet N°5 186

Author's presentation..215

References 216

CLINICAL NUTRITION FOR DISEASES OF THE ESOPHAGUS, STOMACH, AND DUODENUM

Diet therapy is traditionally one of the main methods of treatment and metabolic rehabilitation of patients with diseases of the esophagus, stomach, and duodenum. With proper adapted nutrition, the effect is ensured not only due to the sparing principles of the local mechanical, thermal, and biochemical effects of food on the functional state of the stomach (direct effect), but also the positive effect on the whole organism by changing various types of metabolism, nervous, and humoral regulation.

For decades, diseases of the upper gastrointestinal tract have recommended strict adherence to sparing diets. However, today, the use of new drugs that have both an etiotropic and pathogenetic effect on the course of the disease allows patients to adhere to less strict principles in nutrition, which improves their quality of life. At the same time, teaching patients the principles of clinical nutrition is very important today. Patients should know the principles of clinical nutrition, as well as which foods and dishes have an undesirable effect on gastric secretion and motility.

1.1 Principles of Clinical Nutrition

Clinical nutrition should contribute to a targeted effect on metabolism; it should both heal and prevent the exacerbation of different diseases and metabolic disorders.

- It is necessary to observe the correct diet: eat regularly at the same hours.

- It is necessary to diversify the diet.

- Clinical nutrition should be individualized: not a disease is treated, but a patient.

- The balance of the diet: it is necessary to take into account the calorie content and composition of the main products.

- Proper cooking is needed.

- When compiling an individual diet, it is imperative to take into account concomitant diseases.

- Clinical nutrition most effectively contributes to recovery if it is used in combination with other therapeutic factors such as lifestyle changes, physical activation, the use of mineral waters, dietary supplements, etc.

1.1.1 Effects of Food on Gastric Physiology

1.1.1.1 Effects on Gastric Secretion

The effects of food on gastric secretion are different. On this basis, the products are divided into strong and weak secretors.

- The strong secretors include foods containing extractive substances (meat, fish, mushroom broths, strong navar from vegetables); spices (mustard, cinnamon, horseradish, etc.); fried foods, canned food, tomato sauces, meat and fish stewed in own juice; salted and smoked meat and fish products; salted, pickled vegetables, and fruits; hard-boiled eggs, especially yolks; rye bread and pastry; stale or overheated edible fats; fermented milk products with high acidity, skim milk, whey; strong tea, coffee; drinks containing alcohol; drinks containing carbon dioxide (carbonated); sour and insufficiently ripe fruits, berries, and raw vegetables.

- A weak stimulating effect on gastric secretion is inherent in: drinking water; dairy products (skim milk, cream, cottage cheese); starch; soft-boiled eggs or as an omelet; well-boiled meat and boiled fresh fish; mashed vegetables; fats; dairy or mucous soups of cereals and vegetables (potatoes, carrots, and beets); sweet fruit puree; dishes of semolina and boiled rice, liquid milk porridges; yesterday's white bread; alkaline waters that do not contain carbon dioxide; weak tea.

- Fats have a biphasic effect on gastric secretion. Initially, fats suppress gastric secretion, and later on, saponification products of fats formed in the intestines stimulate gastric secretion.

- An important role is played by the culinary processing of food. Fried meat is a stronger stimulant of gastric secretion than boiled meat.

- The consistency of food also affects gastric secretion. A piece of meat is a stronger stimulator of gastric secretion than meat soufflé since it does not evacuate from the stomach for longer. The gruel and liquid food are more quickly removed from the stomach.

- With a combination of food products, their effect on gastric secretion changes somewhat. For example, the addition of fats to proteins reduces gastric hypersecretion but lengthens its time.

1.1.1.2 Effects on Gastric Motility

The effect of food on the motor function of the stomach depends, first of all, on its consistency and composition. Solid food is evacuated from the stomach later than gruel. The fastest carbohydrates are evacuated from the stomach, the proteins are somewhat slower, and the fats are the last.

1.2 Basics of Clinical Nutrition for Diseases of the Esophagus, Stomach, and Duodenum

Diet therapy of diseases of the upper digestive tract takes into account the basic and most important principles of mechanical, biochemical, and thermal sparing. Sparing diets include primarily foods that are weak stimulators of gastric secretions, quickly leaving the stomach and not irritating its mucous membrane. Regular and fractional nutrition, which facilitates the conditions of digestion and assimilation of food, also contributes to the sparing regime of the functioning of the stomach.

- The mechanical irritation of the gastric mucosa is promoted by a large amount of food administered at one meal; intake of foods rich in coarse fiber (radish, turnips, beans, peas with husks, unripe fruits, gooseberries, grapes, raisins, currants, dates, and whole meal bread); intake of foods rich in connective tissue (cartilage, sinewy meat, poultry, and fish skin).

- Chemical irritation of the mucous membrane of the digestive tract is exerted by foods and dishes that have an aggressive chemical environment (acidic or alkaline), as well as substances that strongly stimulate gastric secretion.

- The thermal effect on the mucous membrane of the stomach has a very cold and hot food.

- The gentle principle of building therapeutic diets provides for a gradual transition from one diet to another, taking into account the nature, form, stage of the disease, and possible complications and the condition of other organs of the digestive system.

1.2.1 Diseases of the Esophagus

1.2.1.1 Gastroesophageal Reflux Disease

Gastroesophageal reflux disease (GERD) refers to a group of diseases with primary motor impairment. This term refers to all cases of pathological reflux of the acidic contents of the stomach into the esophagus with a drop in pH in the lumen of the esophagus below 4.0 (normal 5.5-7). In the primary prevention and treatment of this disease, an important role is played by proper nutrition, as well as a change in the patient's lifestyle.

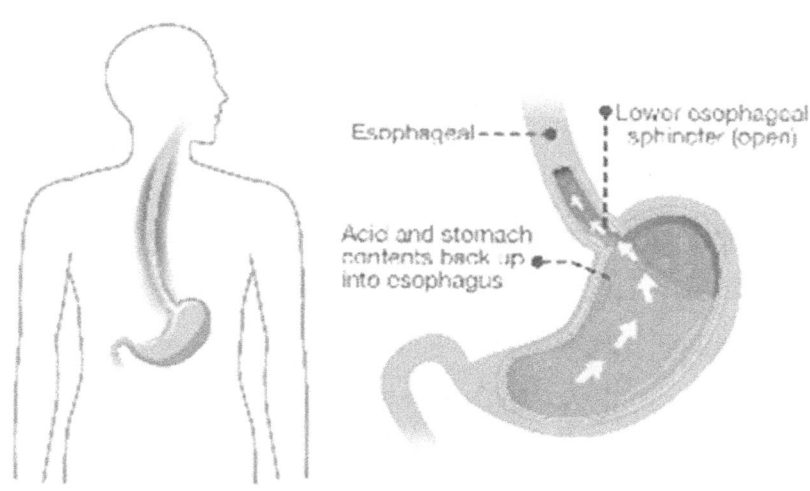

1.2.1.1.1 Lifestyle recommendations

- Stop smoking.

- Normalize body weight.

- Avoid stress on the abdominal muscles, work incline, and wearing tight belts.

- Sleep on a bed whose head-end is raised 10-15 cm (especially if symptoms occur at night).

- Control the intake of drugs that can inhibit the motility of the esophagus and the function of the lower esophageal sphincter or have a direct damaging effect on the mucous membrane of the esophagus.

- Normalize the stool.

1.2.1.1.2 Nutritional Recommendations

- Exclude overeating and snacks before bedtime. The last meal no later than 2 hours before bedtime.

- Do not lie down after meals for 2 hours.

- Eat 3-4 times a day in small portions.

- Stop drinking alcohol.

- Exclude hot, very cold, and spicy food from the diet; they have a damaging effect on the mucous membrane of the esophagus.

- Exclude carbonated drinks that increase intragastric pressure and thereby contribute to gastroesophageal reflux.

- Eliminate or reduce the intake of fats, which inhibit the motor activity of the stomach.

- Limit or exclude the use of foods that contribute to hypotension of the lower esophageal sphincter - coffee, chocolate, green onions and garlic, tomatoes, and citrus fruits.

There is no special diet for patients with GERD. Perhaps the use of Diet N°1 could be adequate.

In overweight patients who abuse smoking, alcohol, as well as those who do not comply with dietary and lifestyle changes, the course of the disease is refractory to treatment.

1.2.1.2 Achalasia of the Cardia

Achalasia of the cardia is a chronic neuromuscular disease in which the passage of food goes through the esophagus, and from the esophagus to the stomach, it is disturbed due to pathological changes in the esophageal peristalsis and the absence of reflex relaxation of the lower esophageal sphincter during swallowing.

1.2.1.2.1 Nutritional Recommendations

Frequent (5-6 times a day) meal;

- Moderately sparing diet: avoid spicy, oily, and hot food.

- Exclude alcohol.

- In the formation of protein-energy deficiency, artificial nutrition is indicated.

1.2.1.3 Esophagospasm

Esophagospasm is a disease characterized by occasionally occurring spastic contractions of the esophagus wall, which is based on a violation of the primary and secondary peristalsis of the thoracic esophagus, mainly of hypermotor nature.

1.2.1.3.1 Nutritional Recommendantions

- Regular nutrition (5-6 times a day) is of great importance.

- The predominant use of liquid or gruel-like food.

- With secondary (reflex) esophagospasm, a moderately sparing diet is needed to prevent mechanical, thermal, and chemical irritating effects on the mucous membrane of the esophagus. Exclusion from the diet of cold and hot foods, carbonated drinks, acidic foods, foods containing coarse fiber (cabbage, apples, etc.), fresh pastries,, and bread.

- Exclude alcohol.

1.2.2 Diseases of the Stomach and Duodenum

1.2.2.1 Functional Dyspepsia

Functional dyspepsia is a symptom complex of functional disorders, including pain or discomfort in the epigastric region, heaviness, a feeling of fullness after eating, early satiety, bloating, nausea, vomiting, belching, heartburn, and other signs in which it is not possible to detect organic diseases. An important place in the treatment of patients with functional dyspepsia is diet therapy. With functional dyspepsia, a balanced diet is recommended; strictly restrictive diets should not be followed.

1.2.2.1.1 Nutritional Recommendations

- Frequent fractional nutrition is needed. Patients should avoid long breaks in food intake. Dietary intake should be fractionated, 5-6 times a day.

- The food should be moderately hot, and its preliminary grinding is not required.

- Indigestible and coarse foods are excluded from the diet.

- A highly specific response in the form of dyspepsia to fat intake has been proven in clinical studies. Patients noted symptoms of dyspepsia after eating a meal rich in fat, but in cases where the fat was hidden, the food was well tolerated. In addition, the consistency of the food and the method of its culinary processing mattered. For example, dyspepsia was less likely to occur after eating fat-containing solid foods than fat-containing fluids. Adding margarine to liquid foods significantly exacerbates the symptoms of dyspepsia. In this regard, with functional dyspepsia, it is recommended to limit the free fat rate in the diet.

- Patients with a dyskinetic variant of the disease should avoid products that have an irritating effect on the gastric mucosa: strong broths, smoked meats, canned foods, hot spices and spices, black coffee, strong tea, and carbonated drinks.

- With an ulcer-like variant of dyspepsia, the use of strong stimulants of gastric secretion (strong broths and broths, coffee, cocoa, carbonated drinks, marinades, etc.) is not recommended. If hypersecretion of the stomach is based on the increased excitability of the autonomic nervous system, then it is recommended to limit the amount of carbohydrates to 150-200g per day.

- A sufficient amount of vitamin B1 (thiamine) must be supplied with the diet, which stimulates the tone and motility of the gastrointestinal tract.

- All patients with dyspepsia should cease smoking.

- A ban on alcohol abuse is needed.

- Stop taking NSAIDs.

1.2.2.2 Acute Gastritis

Treatment of acute gastritis should begin with the causes of the disease. In some cases, the main thing in emergency care should be gastric lavage. The stomach is recommended to be washed with isotonic sodium chloride solution, 0.5% sodium bicarbonate solution (1 tsp. Baking soda per 1 liter of water), mineral or ordinary warm water. For the complete release of the gastrointestinal tract from damaging factors, it is possible to use a cleansing enema. After washing the stomach, the patient is prescribed bed rest for 2-3 days.

1.2.2.2.1 Nutritional Recommendations

- At the beginning of the development of the disease, complete fasting is recommended. During the first 1-2 days, it is recommended to refrain from eating completely. Of the drinks, strong tea, warm alkaline mineral water such as borzhoma, unsweetened dried fruit compote are allowed in small portions at this time. Drinking should be warm, with a volume of 1-1.5 liters per day.

- Then a low caloric diet is introduced for 1-2 days.

- After 2-3 days from the onset of the disease, diet N°1a is allowed.

- After 4 days, diet N°1b is prescribed.

- This is followed by diet N°1.

- After 6-8 days, the patient is transferred to normal balanced diet.

Preventive measures to prevent the development of chronic gastritis are reduced to the observance of a balanced diet (no indigestible, hot food, spicy seasonings), no of abuse alcohol, and smoking.

Within 6 months, as a metabolic rehabilitation measure, it is recommended to fortify the patient's diet, especially with vitamins such as C, A, and PP.

Failure to follow metabolic rehabilitation measures, indulging in one's addictions leads to the transition of the disease into a chronic form, the development of chronic gastritis or even peptic ulcer.

1.2.2.3 Chronic Gastritis

Diet therapy of chronic gastritis depends on the type of secretory function impairment (gastritis with preserved and increased secretory activity of secretory insufficiency), the phase of the disease (exacerbation, remission) and its form, as well as the severity of pathological changes in the stomach and concomitant damage to organs and systems.

When choosing a diet, the following should be taken into account: the nature of secretory disorders (preserved or increased secretion; secretory insufficiency - moderate, severe); individual tolerance of certain dishes; complete and balanced diet; the severity and activity of the inflammatory process in the gastric mucosa.

Clinical nutrition differs significantly in chronic gastritis with preserved (and increased) secretion from dietary recommendations in chronic gastritis with secretory insufficiency. But at the same time, clinical nutrition for chronic gastritis should be optimized for a sick person and fully satisfy his physiological need for food ingredients.

It should be noted that for a short time with a pronounced exacerbation of chronic gastritis, it is recommended to use physiologically defective "hungry" diets. The need for their use is due to a pronounced violation of the functions of the digestive tract. In such cases, the weight of the daily ration is reduced, and liquid and gruel-like food are prescribed, which has the least mechanical effect on the stomach.

In chronic gastritis, patients should receive more than previously recommended in diet N°1, the amount of dietary fiber in the form of heat-treated or raw vegetables and fruits. This helps to normalize the intestinal passage, improve digestion and metabolism, and helps to relieve the symptoms of colon dysbiosis.

With pronounced fermentation processes, it is necessary to limit carbohydrates. It is important to enrich the diet with vitamins due to the deterioration of their resorption.

With a reduced diet, it is necessary to increase the energy value of the diet, especially due to protein. With the development of anemia, it is necessary to enrich the diet with salts of iron, copper and vitamins (especially ascorbic acid, thiamine, and cobalamin).

Currently, in hospitals, in the treatment of chronic gastritis, it is recommended to use a well-balanced standard diet.

1.2.2.3.1 Nutritional Recommendations for Chronic Atrophic Gastritis (with secretory insufficiency)

With chronic atrophic gastritis (with secretory insufficiency), clinical nutrition is aimed at reducing inflammatory changes in the gastric mucosa, stimulating its glandular apparatus, as well as increasing the compensatory capabilities of other digestive organs.

In the exacerbation phase, it is necessary to assign a diet variant with mechanical and biochemical sparing for 5-7 days. It is possible to recommend diet N°1a, which provides the gentle principle of mechanical and thermal effects on the stomach. Eating in a warm, well-cooked form provides a gentle principle of thermal and mechanical influence on the function of the stomach and helps to reduce inflammation. Adequate food chopping improves enzymatic digestion and assimilation.

With moderate exacerbation, it is possible to introduce mild chemical stimulants of gastric secretion (tea, cocoa, weak coffee, fruit and vegetable juices, low-fat broths from meat, poultry and fish, and soups made from fresh vegetables). The introduction of chemical irritants stimulates the secret function of the stomach. Patients are further recommended diet N°2 (in the absence of concomitant damage to the liver, biliary tract, and pancreas). This is a physiologically complete diet with moderate mechanical grinding of food and moderate stimulation of the secretion of digestive organs.

In the phase of remission of chronic atrophic gastritis, the diet, as a rule, should not be too sparing. Mechanically ground food contributes to constipation. An increase in appetite is provided by cabbage, onions, cucumbers, parsley, radish, dill, horseradish, garlic, quince, lingonberries, cherries, pomegranates, strawberries, strawberries, raspberries, mountain ash, red and black currants. Perhaps the use of special "mouth-watering" herbal teas. The sokogonny effect of vegetables is somewhat reduced after cooking.

In chronic gastritis with secretory insufficiency with a tendency to diarrhea in the acute stage, diet N°4b is recommended, after which diet N°4c is used. Food on this diet contains relatively few carbohydrates and, therefore, less calories. Coarse vegetable fibers, whole milk, first and second courses in milk, salt, and spices, depending on the condition of the patient, are limited or completely excluded. In addition, very cold and hot dishes are excluded. On a set of diet products, diet N°4 is full. All dishes should be boiled or steamed - desirable infusions and jelly from blueberries or black currants. Raw vegetables and fruits, nuts, brown bread, fresh berries, and canned food are completely excluded from the diet.

Often with chronic atrophic gastritis, the liver, pancreas, gall bladder are involved in the pathological process. In such cases, the purpose of diet N°5a (with the exception of pure milk) or diet N°4b, which is replaced by diet N°4c or diet N°5, is indicated.

With concomitant inflammation of the pancreas (pancreatitis), carbohydrates are reduced in the diet (up to 300-500g per day), and the protein content is increased (up to 140-160g per day).

The most acceptable diet for most patients with chronic gastritis in the phase of persistent remission is a well-balanced standard diet, which provides the body's needs for basic food products and their sufficient digestibility. Standard diet should contain a balanced amount of proteins, fats, carbohydrates and minerals, and an increased amount of vitamins, which allows to use a variety of culinary processing of products.

Most patients with chronic atrophic gastritis do not tolerate whole milk, which causes flatulence, air belching, and stool disorder. In these cases, milk should be excluded from the diet. In such cases, it is better to use fermented milk products (kefir, yogurt), cottage cheese (fresh or in the form of casseroles, pudding).

With a prolonged course of chronic gastritis with secretory insufficiency, iron deficiency anemia and enteritis usually develop, so the additional intake of nutrients into the patient's body is very important. The diet is enriched with protein, vitamins, and iron. In addition, with enteritis, products containing a large amount of phosphorus and calcium should also be added to the patient's menu.

In chronic atrophic gastritis, N Acetyl Cysteine can be prescribed at a dose of 1-1.5g/day for 24-25 days. It has a pronounced potentiating effect on the parietal cells of the gastric glands, prolonging their action up to 2–2.5 hours. Cysteine, which is part of the drug, is converted to glutathione, which has a mainly peripheral effect on parietal cells. It is completely harmless and free from side effects.

Currently, in the treatment of chronic gastritis, it is recommended to use a standard well-balanced diet.

1.2.2.3.2 Nutritional Recommendations for Chronic Gastritis with preserved (and increased) secretion

With exacerbation of chronic gastritis with normal or increased secretion in the first 1-2 days, it is recommended to refrain from eating, plenty of water is allowed.

Next, the patient is assigned a diet N°1a with mechanical and biochemical sparing. This diet is usually prescribed for 1-3 days, less often 3-5 days. The diet must be fractionated to 5-6 times a day. 7-10 days after diet N°1a, diet N°1b is prescribed. It is prescribed for 1-2 weeks.

As the exacerbation subsides, depending on the type of secretory disorders, the diet differentiates.

With a positive dynamics of pain and dyspeptic syndromes (in the absence of nausea, belching, heartburn), diet N°1 is recommended, which patients with chronic gastritis should adhere to for several months. From the diet, exclude products and dishes with irritating effects.

The next stage is the transition to diet N°5. This diet stimulates bile secretion and intestinal motility. The timing of the use of a particular diet is selected individually and depends on the characteristics of the course of the disease. From the patient's diet for a long period (even after the onset of persistent remission), it is recommended to exclude products that strongly excite gastric secretion: essential oils, organic acids, and extractive substances of meat and fish.

With persistent remission, the diet is gradually expanded, trying to get closer to a balanced diet, except for strong chemical irritants of the gastric mucosa and gastric secretion stimulants.

1.2.2.3.3 Mineral Waters for Chronic Gastritis.

The course of dietary treatment of chronic gastritis is long and ranges from several months to 2-3 years. As a metabolic rehabilitation measure, a spa treatment is prescribed. A prerequisite for its implementation is a stable remission.

Mineral waters contribute to the elimination of the inflammatory process in the gastric mucosa and the elimination of its functional disorders. Drinking a course of mineral waters has a restorative effect on the body, positively affects the functional state of other digestive organs and the defeat of which often accompanies chronic gastritis.

As a rule, more mineralized waters (more than 600 mg/l of dry residues) can stimulate the secretory function of the stomach, and less mineralized ones (less than 300 mg/l of dry residues) tend to moderately inhibit the secretory activity of the gastric glands.

In the case of secretory insufficiency, it is recommended to use water from salt-alkaline sources 15–20 minutes before a meal, and with preserved and increased secretory function, it is bicarbonate 1 hour before a meal and during heartburn.

The dosage of mineral waters is strictly individual.

The duration of treatment with water is 3-4 weeks or more.

1.2.2.4 Peptic Ulcer

Clinical nutrition traditionally plays a large role in the treatment of peptic ulcers. Despite the increase in the effectiveness of modern drug treatment for peptic ulcers, diet therapy has not lost its significance in our time. Helicobacter pylori eradication alone in case of peptic ulcer will not be able to restore the functions of the gastrointestinal tract quickly; therefore, all patients are advised to follow the developed regimes of clinical nutrition, especially for prolonged and severe peptic ulcer disease.

The principle of individualization of diet therapy is to select the diet of patients for the impact of its components on the main pathogenetic mechanisms of development and chronicity of the disease, taking into account the phase of the pathological process, gender, age, and dietary inclinations of the patient.

Diet therapy should take into account the phase of the course of peptic ulcer (acute, subacute, and incomplete remission), clinical and pathogenetic features of the disease (localization of peptic ulcer), and the presence of complications and associated pathology.

The purpose of clinical nutrition for peptic ulcer disease: creating favorable conditions for the elimination of pain, dyspeptic complaints, and healing of ulcers. This is achieved by prescribing a therapeutic diet devoid of irritating effects on the stomach, which meets the gentle principles of biochemical and thermal effects on the mucous membrane of the stomach and duodenum. The diet can reduce the activity of the acid-peptic factor due to the buffering properties of food ingredients, to reduce the reflex excitability of the stomach and duodenum, and to stimulate the processes of physiological and reparative regeneration.

1.2.2.4.1 Nutritional Recommendations in the Acute Phase of Recurrence of Peptic Ulcer

In the acute phase of peptic ulcer disease, it is necessary to ensure maximum digestive system sparing. Functional gastric sparing is achieved due to fractional nutrition, the nature of the mechanical processing of food (crushed, jelly-like or puree, gruel-like), and restrictions on the diet of easily digestible carbohydrates (sugar and sugar-containing products). The correct rhythm of nutrition is of great importance. A meal is recommended every 3-4 hours, in small portions.

It is important to eliminate the existing deficiency of vitamins due to ascorbic acid, riboflavin, and pyridoxine, which stimulate regeneration processes; retinol, promoting ulcer epithelization; thiamine, eliminating trophic disorders; the routine that strengthens the vascular wall.

Clinical nutrition in the acute phase of relapse, with severe pain;

In the period of severe exacerbation of gastric ulcer and duodenal ulcer with characteristic symptoms of an irritated stomach, it is recommended to use diet N°1a (as sparing as possible) - for the first 3-5 days of treatment.

Diet N°1a provides for eating in liquid, gruel and jelly-like form. Such nutrition helps to accelerate the repair of ulcers and erosion, as well reduce the activity of the inflammatory process of the mucous membrane of the upper gastrointestinal tract. The purpose of this diet is to normalize the healing processes of the mucous membrane and reduce the effect of aggressive, irritating agents on the receptor apparatus of the stomach and duodenum, as well as regulate the secretory and motor-evacuation functions of the stomach, and reduce the excitability of the autonomic nervous system. Diet N°1a fully provides the physiological needs of the body for nutrients and trace elements in strict bed rest.

1.2.2.4.2 Nutritional Recommendations in the Subacute Phase of Recurrence of Peptic Ulcer

In the subacute phase of the recurrence of peptic ulcer (the next 5–7 days), they switch to food according to the principles of diet N°1b (a more stressful diet). The difference from diet N°1a is a gradual increase in the content of basic nutrients and caloric intake.

Diet N°1b is also used subject to bed rest. With positive clinical dynamics, a quick transition is possible, and sometimes the original purpose of diet N°1 is also possible. Indication for the use of diet N°1: peptic ulcer of the stomach and duodenum during the subsidence of exacerbation.

With the satisfactory well-being of the patient after 2-3 weeks, a transition to a standard diet is recommended.

When in a hospital, patients with peptic ulcer in the exacerbation phase are assigned a diet option with mechanical and biochemical sparing, and in remission, a standard well-balanced diet.

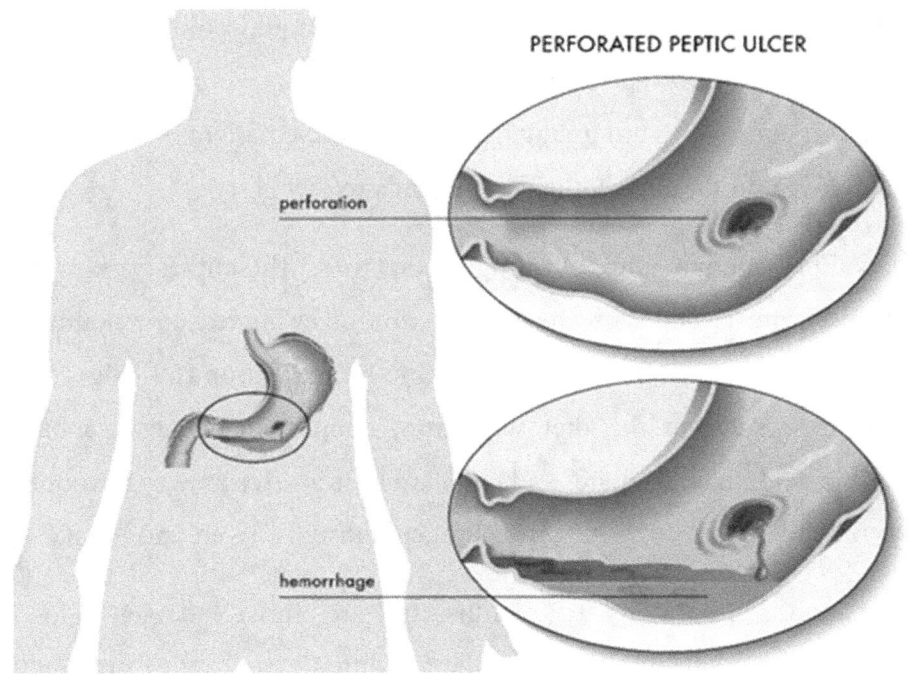

1.2.2.5 Complicated Course of Peptic Ulcer

1.2.2.5.1 Nutrition for long-term ulcerative ulcers

Poor, prolonged healing of ulcers, marked concomitant diseases, the presence of protein-energy deficiency requires an increase in the diet of protein, carbohydrates, and vitamins. In this regard, whenever possible, one should reduce the length of stay on diets N°1a and N°1b and balance them with diet N°1c.

1.2.2.5.2 Food for Ulcerative Bleeding

For ulcerative bleeding, a specialized diet should be used. To the complete cessation of bleeding, the patient, if indicated, receives parenteral nutrition.

After the cancellation of parenteral nutrition, liquid cold food (milk, jelly, cream) is allowed (200 ml/day), and then sour cream, raw eggs, butter, mucous soups are gradually added, and the patient is transferred to diet N°1a. In the future, the diet expands to diet N°1.

To combat anemia after bleeding, a diet of sufficient energy value should be prescribed with the introduction of an increased amount of high-grade proteins (140–150g) and some fat restriction (60–70g). It is necessary to enrich the diet with iron, copper, manganese, cobalt, ascorbic acid, niacin, folate, and cobalamin. It is advisable to introduce into the diet dishes containing hematogen nutrients, liver, and yeast.

With good health, after 1-1.5 months, they are allowed to use the food in the unground form with the addition of raw fruits and vegetables. Sweet soft fruits (plums, apples, etc.) and vegetables can also be consumed in non-mashed form. Then they gradually switch to a balanced diet; however, one should keep in mind the need to observe regularity in nutrition and caution when consuming spicy, rough, too hot, cold food, and alcohol.

1.2.2.5.3 Nutrition for Stenosis of the Outlet of the Stomach

With a complication of peptic ulcer, stenosis of the outlet of the stomach in connection with the developing depletion of the body shows an increase in the energy value of the diet due to an increase in the quantity of high-grade proteins and enrichment with vitamins.

It is especially important to introduce an increased amount of thiamine, which stimulates the motor activity of the stomach and promotes its emptying.

Violation of the evacuation function of the stomach determines the need to increase the interval between meals and reduce the amount administered at one meal. Food is used in liquid and semi-liquid form.

With repeated vomiting, the threat of dehydration requires the use of an increased amount of salt and a sufficient amount of liquid (preferably in the form of fruit and vegetable juices), which are recommended to be taken separately from solid food (after 2-3 hours).

In severe cases, additional parenteral administration of a liquid (5% glucose solution) and especially saline solutions (sodium chloride solutions) are indicated. Patients can be fed enteral mixtures for a long time both orally and by creating enteral access. In some cases, the use of parenteral nutrition is necessary.

1.2.2.6 Stomach Cancer

Information on the effect of food on the growth and development of malignant tumors is still limited. Experimental and some clinical observations suggest a stimulating effect on malignant growth and metastasis of nutrition with high energy value, use of high amounts of cholesterol-rich fats and a limited protein intake, high doses of alpha tocopherol and small doses of retinol, excessive administration of simple carbohydrates and other toxic substances such as pesticides, pollutants and synthetic molecules. Diets with a high content of protein, choline and limited content of trans fats, as well as the use of pyridoxine, folate, and niacin, large doses of retinol, iodine, zinc, and phosphorus, have an inhibitory effect on the growth of malignant tumors in general. As cancer is a very complex disease, there are exceptions and contradictions depending on the micronutrients and molecules, the circumstances of their use, the type of cancer and the metabolism of the patient.

With timely recognition of gastric cancer, radical surgical treatment is indicated. In inoperable cases, in order to delay the growth and metastasis of the tumor, it is recommended to use diets with a moderate energy value, rich in proteins, vitamins (retinol, ascorbic acid, riboflavin, pyridoxine, niacin, and folate), methionine, choline, calcium, iodine, iron, zinc, phosphorus, a restriction of simple carbohydrates, and animal fats rich in cholesterol.

Dysphagia in cancer of the cardiac part of the stomach is facilitated by the appointment of liquid and jelly-like dishes (kefir, beaten eggs, jelly, fruit and milk jelly, cocoa, coffee, broth, etc.), taking 1-2 tablespoons of sunflower oil in 20-30 minutes before meals. When stenosis of the pyloric part of the stomach, food should be consumed in small portions in liquid and mushy form. With severe stenosis, parenteral nutrition is indicated.

In case of obstruction of solid food during stenosis of the cardiac part of the stomach and esophagus, it is advisable to eat enteral mixtures orally. With severe stenosis, enteral nutrition through a gastrostomy is advisable, and if formation is not possible, parenteral nutrition.

Pain and dyspeptic disorders associated with concomitant gastritis and ulceration due to tumor decay can be somewhat relieved by the use of sparing diets used in chronic gastritis and peptic ulcer disease.

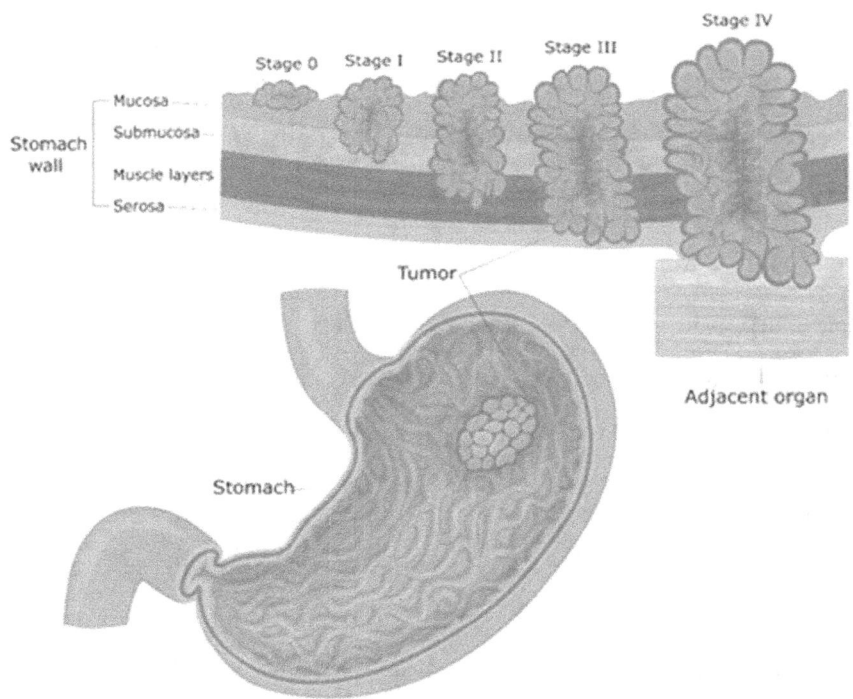

CLINICAL NUTRITION FOR DISEASES OF THE LIVER AND BILIARY TRACT

Chronic diseases of the liver and biliary tract occur in most cases as a result of acute infections or as a result of prolonged alcohol abuse, especially against the background of a disordered diet and lack of protein products and vitamins in the diet, as well as metabolic disorders (gallstone disease) and congenital genetic defects.

Among acute liver diseases, acute viral hepatitis and acute cholecystitis (or exacerbation of chronic cholecystitis) are most common. The most common forms of chronic liver damage are chronic hepatitis and chronic cholecystitis.

The occurrence of exacerbations of diseases is facilitated by colds, various infections, cooling, overwork, and prolonged severe eating disorders (alcohol abuse, overeating, especially fatty, spicy, smoked and salty foods, as well as foods rich in cholesterol).

Diet therapy of liver diseases is prescribed by a doctor and is determined depending on the stage of the disease and the condition of the patient. The main diet for patients with diseases of the liver and biliary tract for many decades in our country was diet N°5.

2.1 General Recommendations

When preparing diets for patients with diseases of the liver and biliary tract, the following recommendations should be considered:

- The diet should have a sufficient amount of complete, easily digestible protein.

- The quality and quantity of fat is determined by the condition of the patient. If necessary, enhance the choleretic effect of the diet, the content of vegetable fats increases, especially with constipation.

- The amount of carbohydrates in the diet should not exceed the physiological norm, and in patients with overweight, it can be reduced.

- The maximum sparing of the patient's digestive tract is achieved by culinary processing of food (boiled, chopped or mashed food, if necessary).

- Frequent fractional nutrition, which provides better digestion and assimilation of food, has a good choleretic effect and improves intestinal motility.

- The inclusion in the diet of foods rich in dietary fiber, which increases the choleretic effect of the diet, provides maximum excretion of cholesterol with stool.

In recent years, diet N°5 has undergone a number of changes, its modifications have been developed, but the principles of its compilation have remained relevant until now.

The energy value of the diet for patients with diseases of the liver and biliary tract should correspond to the physiological norm, and overeating is not desirable. The amount of proteins in the diet should correspond to the physiological norm: 1g/kg of ideal body weight, of which 50–55% should be proteins of animal origin (meat, fish, poultry, eggs, dairy products).

Animal proteins are rich in essential amino acids and lipotropic factors (methionine, choline), which prevent the development of fatty liver. Of plant products, a large amount of methionine and choline contains soy flour, oat, and buckwheat.

An increased amount of protein (up to 1.5g/kg) is required for patients with alcoholic liver damage and protein-energy deficiency. Limit food proteins in hepatic cell failure, while preferring plant proteins. Diet N°5 includes 70-80g of fat per day. Fats of animal origin should be 2/3, vegetable 1/3 of the total amount of fats.

Limit the total amount of fat in the diet to 50g per day or less only in some cases: with steatorrhea of any genesis (liver, pancreatic, intestinal); with diarrhea; with hepatic cell failure; in the early stages after cholecystectomy.

Increase the total amount of fat to 100-120g due to vegetables, if necessary, enhance the choleretic effect of food. The ratio of animal to vegetable fats is 1:1. A similar diet can be prescribed for about 3 weeks in the presence of extrahepatic cholestasis and constipation.

Of animal fats, it is best to use butter, as it is well absorbed and contains vitamins A, K, and arachidonic acid. It is necessary to limit the consumption of refractory fats (mutton, pork, beef fats) because they are difficult to digest, contain a lot of cholesterol and saturated fatty acids, and can contribute to the formation of cholesterol stones and the development of fatty liver. Adequate use of vegetable oils is very important: sunflower, corn, olive, cotton, and soy. Vegetable oils enhance bile formation and bile secretion by stimulating the synthesis of the hormone cholecystokinin. Unsaturated fatty acids (linoleic, linolenic, arachidonic) activate lipolysis enzymes, improve cholesterol metabolism. In diet N°5, restrict fried foods.

Diet N°5 contains 300–350g of carbohydrates, of which 60–70g is simple. In the standard diet, the amount of carbohydrates is reduced due to simple ones (300–330g in total, 30–40g simple). With excess body weight, the amount of carbohydrates is limited due to mono- and disaccharides. Diets with low energy value, consisting solely of digestible carbohydrates, are prescribed for severe liver failure.

Indigestible carbohydrates play an important role in the diet (see The role of dietary fiber in nutrition) cellulose, hemicellulose, and pectin substances. The main sources of dietary fiber are fruits, berries, vegetables, and bran. When bran is used, the amount of primary increases and the amount of secondary bile acids decreases. This is due to the influence of dietary fiber on the bacterial flora of the intestine, which is involved in the dehydroxylation of primary bile acids. The binding ability of various dietary fibers with respect to bile acids is not the same. It is especially high for fruits (apples, pears), berries (raspberries), vegetables (cauliflower, carrots, potatoes, parsnips, and green peas), wheat bran, and wholemeal bread. Despite the high content of dietary fiber in lettuce, nuts, and beans, these products limit or exclude liver diseases.

Vitamins are of great importance in the nutrition of patients with diseases of the liver and biliary tract. Multivitamin deficiency can develop in patients due to their limited intake with food, insufficient absorption of vitamins from the intestine, as well as the formation of biologically active and transport forms of vitamins in the liver. The most disturbed is the absorption of fat-soluble vitamins (A, D, E, and K) due to the insufficiency of bile acids necessary for their absorption.

The poor tolerance of cold food (ice cream, kefir from the refrigerator, etc.), which can cause spasm of the sphincter of Oddi and pain, up to an attack of hepatic colic, should be emphasized. In diseases of the liver and biliary tract outside the acute phase in hospitals, a basic standard diet is used.

2.2 Acute Cholecystitis, Exacerbation of Chronic Cholecystitis

In the acute period of the disease, the maximum sparing of the gall bladder and digestive organs as a whole is shown. For 1–2 days, the patient is on a hungry diet — he drinks small portions of weak tea with sugar, rosehip broth, juices in half with boiled water (only 2-3 glasses a day).

Then the diet includes sparing carbohydrate foods: mucous soups, mashed soups, liquid mashed cereals from semolina, rice, oatmeal with a small amount of milk, mashed compotes, jelly, sweet berry, and fruit mousses. In the future, with good clinical dynamics, the diet expands due to the addition of low-fat mashed fresh cottage cheese, steamed chopped meat, fish, chicken, boiled fish with a piece, and crackers from white bread. Food is prepared without salt. Patients are fed 5-6 times a day in small portions. The amount of free fluid is 2–2.5 liters. After 5-6 days, diet N°5a is prescribed. When the exacerbation subsides, after 2-3 weeks, diet N°5 is prescribed.

Currently, for use in hospitals, in the first 2-3 weeks of the disease, a diet option with mechanical and biochemical sparing is recommended, and a standard well-balanced diet in the future.

2.3　Chronic Cholecystitis without Exacerbation

The diet should help to reduce the inflammatory process in the gall bladder and bile ducts, improve bile secretion, and normalize the function of the liver, stomach, pancreas, and intestines.

The main diet is diet N°5.

It is possible to make individual changes for special categories of patients. With hyper motor dyskinesia of the gall bladder, spasm of the sphincter of Oddi, non-functioning gall bladder, restriction of fats, egg yolks are shown. In case of hypomotor dyskinesia of the gall bladder, in case of constipation, it is recommended to prescribe a diet with an increased amount of vegetable fats (100–120g/day) for about 3 weeks, enrich the diet with dietary fiber due to vegetables, fruits, berries, and appropriate dietary supplements. In the future, the amount of fat should be brought into line with the physiological norm. Fats should be evenly distributed throughout the day and mixed with food, which contributes to better absorption of fats, optimal bile secretion, and prevents dyspeptic symptoms.

2.4 Gallstone Disease

The emergence of gallstones is facilitated by several nutrition factors: increased energy value of the diet, an excess of flour and cereal dishes, causing a shift in the pH of bile to the acid side, a lack of vegetable oils and vitamin A, and low content of dietary fiber. In the pathogenesis of the formation of cholesterol stones, which occurs in approximately 80% of cases, the role of changes in the composition of bile (increase in cholesterol, decrease in bile acids and lecithin), inflammation of the gall bladder, stagnation of bile and a shift in its pH to the acid side plays a role.

The main role in the occurrence of gallstones belongs to the accelerated synthesis of endogenous cholesterol in the liver. With improper nutrition, there is an increase in the concentration in the bile of secondary bile acids, for example, deoxycholic, which makes bile more lithogenic.

Patients with gallstone disease without exacerbation are prescribed diet N°5, with exacerbation of calculous cholecystitis, diet N°5a. Patients with cholelithiasis are shown to restrict foods rich in cholesterol (offal, eggs, lard). The synthesis of bile acids is improved by protein products (meat, cottage cheese, fish, egg white), and vegetable oils are rich in lecithin, which also has a choleretic effect.

In patients with frequent bouts of hepatic colic, the intake of vegetable oils is limited. Of animal fats, butter is recommended. It is well emulsified and contains vitamins A and K.

To change the reaction of bile to the alkaline side, milk, lactic acid products, cottage cheese, cheese, vegetables (except pumpkin, legumes, and mushrooms), fruits, and berries (except lingonberries and red currants) are prescribed.

In order to reduce the concentration of bile, heavy drinking is shown, drinking water treatment courses with mineral waters.

The diet of patients with biliary tract diseases should contain a sufficient amount of magnesium salts, which reduce spasm of smooth muscles, improve bile secretion, bowel movement and elimination of cholesterol from the body, and have a sedative effect. Wheat bran, buckwheat, millet, watermelon, soy, crabs, and sea kale are the richest in magnesium.

In hospitals, patients with cholelithiasis without exacerbation are prescribed a standard well-balanced diet for exacerbation of calculous cholecystitis - a variant of the diet with mechanical and biochemical sparing.

2.5 Acute Hepatitis

In acute viral hepatitis, clinical nutrition and protective regimen are referred to as basic therapy. For all types of acute viral hepatitis, a diet N°5a is prescribed for 2-6 weeks (sometimes with an unfavorable course of the disease for a longer period). In the future, the transition to diet N°5 for 6-12 months is recommended. With a complete clinical recovery and normalization of laboratory analyses, well-balanced standard nutrition is later recommended.

The diet for acute hepatitis should be physiologically complete, mechanically, biochemically, and thermally sparing, with some restriction of fats and salt, with an increase in free fluid intake up to 2–2.5l in order to detoxify the body. Fruit and berry juices, rosehip broth, weak tea with jam or honey, tea with milk, compotes, and fruit drinks can be taken. In this case, it is necessary to control the amount of fluid administered orally and parenterally and daily diuresis. With signs of fluid retention, the amount of sodium chloride is reduced to 3g per day (dishes are prepared without salt), the liquid is limited at the rate of diuresis of the previous day plus 400 ml.

Diarrhea and steatorrhea in acute hepatitis are an indication for limiting the quota of fats to 50g.

With an aversion to food, nausea, and vomiting, the diet should be based on the individual taste of the patient. The period of refusal of food should not belong.

Patients often prefer a high-carb, low-fat diet (fruits, fruit juices, dairy foods, etc.).

Particular attention in the diet should be given to products with lipotropic effects - these are proteins rich in methionine and choline (cottage cheese, low-fat meat, fish, oatmeal, buckwheat, soy flour, etc.), vegetable oils containing vitamin E, lecithin, and unsaturated fatty acids.

An adequate intake of ascorbic acid and B vitamins (especially B12 and folic acid) is very important.

It is useful to introduce specialized soy protein products rich in essential amino acids, mineral salts, vitamins, phosphatides, and unsaturated fatty acids into the diet of patients.

In hospitals, they are currently using a diet option with mechanical and biochemical sparing. With uncomplicated hepatitis, this diet is prescribed for 4-6 weeks. With an improvement in general condition, the disappearance of jaundice and dyspeptic symptoms, the normalization of the size of the liver and spleen, the patient is recommended the main option of a standard diet. The patient receives the main standard diet for 6–12 months. With a complete clinical recovery and normalization of laboratory data, rational nutrition is recommended.

2.6 Chronic Hepatitis

In the phase of exacerbation of the disease, diet N°5a is usually prescribed, and diet N°5 without exacerbation. With a good general condition of the patient and normal indicators of a laboratory study of liver function, standard nutrition can be recommended only following certain rules.

- Alcoholic beverages should be avoided, as this worsens the prognosis of the disease.

- It is important to eat at certain hours and avoid plentiful meals at night.

- Not shown are products that irritate the mucous membrane of the upper gastrointestinal tract: seasonings, spices, smoked meats, and vegetables rich in essential oils.

- In chronic hepatitis with extrahepatic cholestasis, the quota of vegetable fats is increased to 50% of the total amount of fat.

- With intrahepatic cholestasis, a deficiency of bile salts in the intestinal lumen and skin itching are often observed. Dietary recommendations include adequate intake of proteins and maintaining the proper energy value of the diet.

- In the presence of steatorrhea, the intake of neutral fats, which are poorly tolerated, is not sufficiently absorbed and impair the absorption of calcium, they are limited to 40g/day. An additional source of fat can be triglycerides with an average chain length (coconut oil) of up to 40g/day.

- The patient needs to receive a sufficient amount of calcium by consuming skim milk and cottage cheese, and if necessary, calcium preparations or dietary supplements for food containing calcium.

- In the phase of exacerbation of the disease during inpatient treatment, a diet option with mechanical and biochemical sparing is prescribed, and without exacerbation, a standard well-balanced diet should be recommended.

2.7 Cirrhosis

In the period of compensation of the disease, diet N°5 is recommended.

If the patient is not exhausted, 1g/kg of body weight of proteins is sufficient. A diet enriched with protein (up to 1.5g/kg) is relevant for patients with alcoholic cirrhosis, in the presence of protein-energy deficiency.

With a stable course of cirrhosis and the absence of inclination in laboratory parameters, an additional intake of branched-chain amino acids is not required. Methionine or various other hepatoprotection are not required. Unnecessarily, the proportion of fats in food should not be reduced. Additionally, food should be cooked so that it stimulates appetite. In inpatient treatment, a standard well-balanced diet is used. With the development of complications of cirrhosis of the liver - liver cell failure, portal hypertension, and ascites, appropriate adjustments are made to the diet.

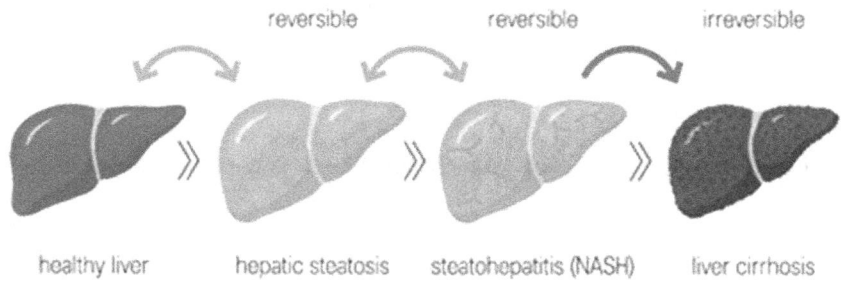

2.8 Hepatic Encephalopathy

One of the main mechanisms of the pathogenesis of hepatic encephalopathy is a violation of the formation of urea from ammonia, which is formed during the deamination of amino acids in the liver. In this case, ammonia penetrates the blood-brain barrier and has a toxic effect on the central nervous system. The main source of amino acids is dietary proteins. That is why it is necessary to reduce protein intake during the development of hepatic encephalopathy to 20 g/day. In acute cases, proteins can be completely excluded from food for a period of several days to several weeks. Even with chronic encephalopathy while limiting the intake of food proteins for several months, clinical signs of protein-energy malnutrition are rare. The energy value of food must be maintained at 1600–2000 kcal or higher.

Parenteral and enteral nutrition, with specialized drugs designed for patients with liver disease, is recommended.

With an improvement in the patient's condition and with a positive dynamics of laboratory parameters, the protein content is increased by 10g every other day. If the recurrence of encephalopathy occurs or laboratory indicators worsen, they return to the previous level of daily protein intake. In patients recovering from an acute episode of coma, the protein content in food is gradually brought back to normal. In chronic encephalopathy, patients need to constantly limit the amount of dietary protein intake to no more than 40-60g/day. Plant proteins are better tolerated than animals. However, eating plant foods can be difficult due to flatulence and diarrhea.

With hepatic encephalopathy, fats are also significantly limited or completely eliminated.

Digestible carbohydrates are administered in sufficient quantities. They recommend fruit and berry juices rich in potassium salts (orange, tangerine, grape, apricot, etc.), dried apricot, apricot, prune infusion, tea with sugar, honey, lemon, jam, and mashed compotes. The total amount of fluid received by the patient is 1.5-2 l/day.

In this case, it is necessary to control the amount of fluid administered orally and parenterally and daily diuresis due to the risk of increasing ascites and edema. With signs of fluid retention, the amount of sodium chloride is reduced to 3g per day (dishes are prepared without salt), the liquid is limited at the rate of diuresis of the previous day plus 400ml.

2.9 Ascites

In patients with ascites, food should receive no more than 22mmol (0.5g) of sodium per day, and the amount of free fluid received should be limited to 1 liter. Failure to follow the recommended diet often leads to the development of poorly treatable ascites. When using more than the permitted amount of salt, even when using diuretic drugs in high doses, treatment may be ineffective.

In ascites, a diet with an energy value of 1,500–2,000kcal is recommended, containing 70g of protein and not more than 22mmol of sodium per day (0.5g). Diet should be essentially vegetarian. Most high protein foods also contain a lot of sodium. The diet needs to be supplemented with low sodium protein foods. Eat salt-free bread and butter. All dishes are prepared without adding salt (diet N°5a in the presence of ascites).

In some cases, with strict observance of the recommended diet, it is possible to quickly achieve a therapeutic effect in patients even without the use of diuretics. These are patients with ascites and edema that first appeared; with normal glomerular filtration rate (creatinine clearance); with reversible liver damage (e.g., fatty liver in alcoholic illness); with acute ascites in infectious disease or bleeding; with ascites that developed after consuming large amounts of sodium (sodium-containing antacids or laxatives, mineral water with high sodium content).

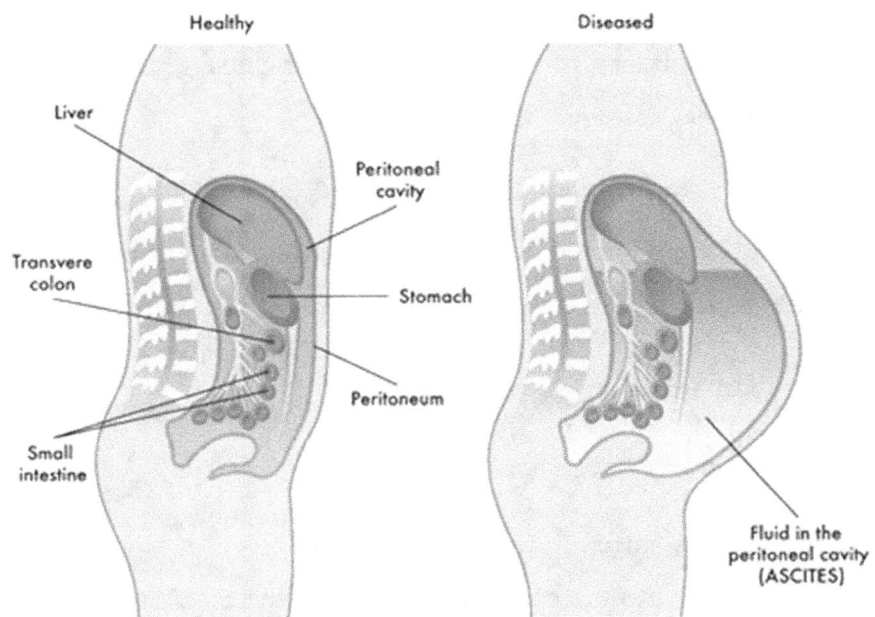

2.10 Alcoholic Liver Disease

In acute alcoholic hepatitis, it is important to quit alcoholic beverages immediately. Diet N°5a is prescribed, and subsequently, diet N°5.

At the initial stage of treatment, the protein content in the daily diet should be 0.5g/kg of body weight, in the future, protein intake is increased to 1g/kg as quickly as possible.

Potassium chloride with magnesium and zinc is added to the food.

High doses of vitamins are prescribed, especially groups B, C, and K (if necessary, intravenously).

Often in alcoholics due to malnutrition, there is a presence of protein-energy deficiency, which helps to reduce immunity, the occurrence of infectious diseases and ascites (due to hypoalbuminemia). In this regard, the importance of good nutrition is obvious, especially in the first days of hospital stay.

The amount of fat in the diet should correspond to the physiological norm, and they are limited only in the presence of steatorrhea, diarrhea, liver failure, and severe dyspeptic syndrome. Fat metabolism disorders are often manifested by hyperlipidemia observed in 30% of alcoholics, and fatty liver, especially in overweight individuals. These conditions require individual correction of the diet.

In some patients suffering from chronic alcoholism, it is necessary to make adjustments to the carbohydrate part of the diet, as depletion of glycogen stores in the liver and a decrease in glucose tolerance may be observed.

In the body of a patient with chronic alcoholism, potassium deficiency is often noted due to poor nutrition and its loss during vomiting and diarrhea. In such cases, additional potassium should be administered with food, and potassium-containing medications should also be prescribed.

Chronic Alcoholism is characterized by zinc deficiency. With proper nutrition, dietary supplements containing zinc are not required, but they are recommended for patients with malnutrition. The following foods are rich in zinc: beef liver, veal, hard cheeses, poultry, shrimp, squid, walnuts, and legumes.

2.11 Wilson – Konovalov's Disease.

In Wilson – Konovalov's disease, there is a genetic defect in the synthesis of ceruloplasmin, which provides copper transport. Decrease or absence of ceruloplasmin disrupts the supply of sufficient amounts of copper to tissue respiration enzymes and blood-forming organs. Free copper accumulating in the tissues is deposited in the liver, brain, kidneys, and cornea.

In Wilson-Konovalov's disease, diet N°5 is prescribed, with limited consumption of products containing copper. It is proved that diet is not of great importance in Wilson-Konovalov disease. However, patients should refrain from eating foods high in copper: chocolate, cocoa, peanuts, mushrooms, legumes, liver, crustaceans, honey, prunes, chestnuts, watercress, lamb, chicken, ducks, and sausages.

Of particular importance is the use of deionized or distilled water if the drinking water contains significant amounts of copper. The use of untested and non-softened water is excluded.

CLINICAL NUTRITION FOR DISEASES OF THE PANCREAS

In recent decades, the incidence of inflammatory, tumor, and other pancreatic diseases has increased significantly. Diseases of the pancreas, in most cases, are quite severe and tend to chronicity. Almost always, chronic pancreatic diseases lead to a significant deterioration in the patient's quality of life.

Clinical nutrition for pancreatic diseases is an integral part of complex therapy. Proper nutrition is necessary in the acute stage of the disease; it helps prevent the progression and chronicity of the disease and compensates for digestive disorders. Thus, clinical nutrition is of great preventive value.

The objectives of diet therapy for pancreatic diseases are correction of the nutritional status of the patient and the elimination of adverse nutritional factors, elimination of body mass deficiency, and symptom of malabsorption.

Dietary recommendations for each specific patient should be made individually, taking into account the type, severity of the disease, food intolerance, concomitant pathology, and taste characteristics.

In clinical nutrition for diseases of the pancreas, strict phasing in expanding the diet is important. The phasing of diet therapy implies a gradual transition from complete hunger in acute pancreatitis (or exacerbation of chronic pancreatitis) to physiologically complete diets.

Compliance with the principles of clinical nutrition allows in some cases to extend the inter-relapse period and prevent the development of severe complications of chronic pancreatitis.

Prevention of exacerbations of chronic pancreatitis is carried out taking into account the etiological factors that occur in a particular patient.

With alcoholic pancreatitis, the main condition for treatment is a complete rejection of the use of alcoholic beverages.

In the case of gallstone disease, it is necessary to constantly follow diet N°5, the use of enzyme preparations, and litholytic therapy for medical reasons.

3.1 Acute Pancreatitis and Exacerbation of Chronic Pancreatitis

In the treatment of acute pancreatitis and the presence of a pronounced exacerbation of chronic pancreatitis, when there is intense pain, high enzyme and amylazuria, an important goal of treatment is to immobilize the production of pancreatic juice. This goal can be achieved by refusing to eat in solid or liquid form and strict bed rest. It excludes even exposure to the diseased look and smell of food.

There are various opinions regarding the nature of fasting. Some authors consider it necessary to exclude the intake of not only food but also liquids. According to the recommendations of other scientists, patients are allowed to take up to 1.5–2 liters of liquid per day in the form of boiled water, weak tea without sugar, alkaline mineral water without gas, decoction of rose hips (10g per 200 ml).

With severe nutritional disorders from the 2nd day of fasting, as well as with prolonged fasting to compensate for the patient's need for nutrients, patients are prescribed parenteral nutrition.

Depending on the type and severity of the disease, hunger is prescribed for a period of 1-3 to 10-20 days. When determining the terms, it should be remembered that hypercatabolism that develops with prolonged starvation causes the patient to be depleted, slow the reparative processes in the pancreas, and worsen the course of the disease. Therefore, the transition to natural nutrition should be carried out as soon as possible.

The basic principle of nutrition is a careful chylomicrons' gradual expansion of the diet and a slow increase in the amount of food administered.

Use mechanically, thermally, and biochemically sparing diets. All food is steamed or boiled. The food should be liquid or semi-liquid consistency, warm (temperature of ready meals 20–52 ° C). Frequent

(6-8 times/day) meals are recommended in small portions (not more than 300g). In the initial period of treatment after complete hunger, predominantly carbohydrate nutrition (high molecular weight polysaccharides) is prescribed - the first version of diet N°5c.

Further, when the exacerbations subside, food containing a large quantity of easily digestible forms of protein is added to the diet - the second version of the diet N°5c. This diet is balanced and complete in relation to essential nutrients, satisfies the patient's needs for proteins, fats, carbohydrates, vitamins, minerals, and energy.

The diet is widely used animal and vegetable products containing "proteolytic enzyme inhibitors": egg white, oatmeal, soybeans, and potatoes. Given the existing connection between the development and maintenance of pain with a lack of pancreatic enzymes in the duodenum, when the patient begins to eat, he is recommended to take multienzyme preparations inadequate doses with food.

With good tolerance of the second variant of diet N°5c, an additional quota of fats is added to the patient's diet. Due to the pronounced steatorrhea characteristic of pancreatic diseases, it is advisable to make up for losses by enriching the diet with foods containing medium-chain fatty acids (vegetable oils). Patients with steatorrhea and weight loss who are not helped by multienzyme replacement therapy are recommended fats containing short-chain fatty acids (coconut oil) because they are more rapidly hydrolyzed and absorbed, and are well tolerated. However, in 25% of patients, they cause nausea and increase diarrhea.

Refractory fats (especially of animal origin) are poorly tolerated by patients; they support the inflammatory process, increase stomach pain and diarrhea.

Patients are categorically contraindicated products that have a "juice" effect: meat, fish, bone, mushroom broths and decoctions, dishes and products prepared by roasting, etc.

A fundamental measure is the absolute rejection of alcoholic beverages since alcohol is a direct stimulant of pancreatic secretion. Alcohol also has a negative effect on organs and structures associated with the pancreas: stomach, duodenum, sphincter of Oddi, and blood vessels.

Currently, a diet option with mechanical and biochemical sparing is recommended for use in hospitals.

Diet therapy is prescribed for a long period (at least 2-3 months) in order to stimulate metabolic and reparative processes in the pancreas and other organs and systems of the body and normalization of the immune status.

ACUTE PANCREATITIS

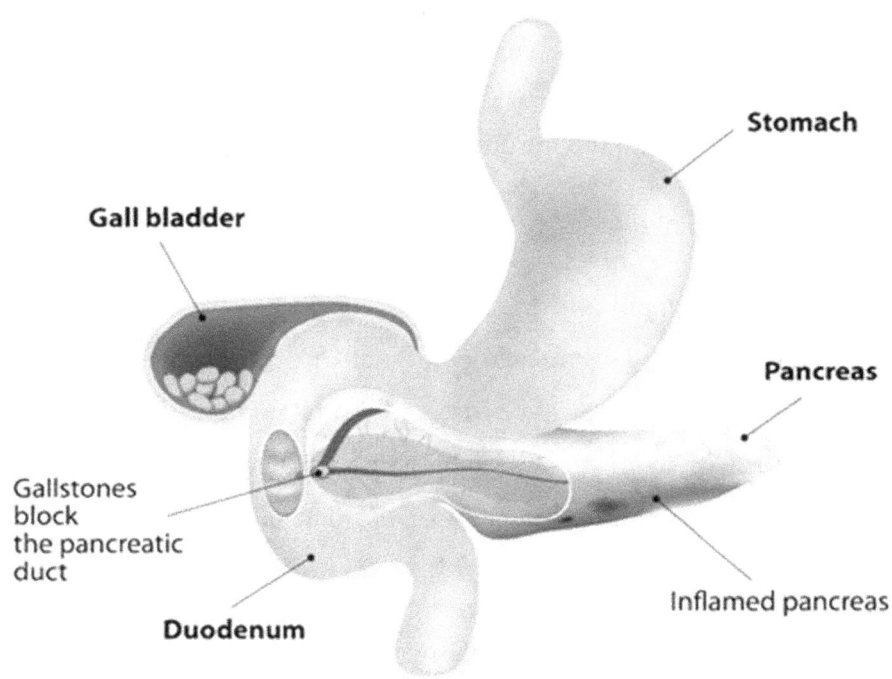

3.2 Remission Phase of Acute and Chronic Pancreatitis

When achieving remission with exacerbation of pancreatitis, it is important to prevent the development of relapses and the progression of pancreatitis, as well as to correct the nutritional disorders that have arisen.

K. Morgenroth et al. (1991), proposed the following dietary regimen for chronic pancreatitis in remission:

- Frequent food intake with a total energy value of 2500-3000 kcal against the background of adequate enzyme therapy.

- Decrease in the amount of fat to 60g/day (540 kcal).

- Carbohydrate intake - 300-400g/day (1200-1600 kcal), if necessary, with the introduction of an adequate dose of insulin.

- Protein intake is 60–120g/day (320–480 kcal).

The long-term appointment of diet N°5 is recommended. In the composition of this daily diet, the amount of proteins corresponds to the physiological needs of the body, and the fat content is increased to 80–90g (30% of them are vegetable), the quota of carbohydrates is 350–400g and the energy intensity of the diet does not exceed 3000 kcal.

During remission, the range of recommended foods and dishes expands. In the phase of remission of chronic pancreatitis, the active inclusion in the diet of various vegetables and fruits in raw, boiled, baked and stewed form is shown. Vegetables are used as part of salads, vinaigrettes, side dishes and as separate dishes. Assigned dishes from various cereals (cereals, pilaf with dried fruits, carrots and boiled meat, puddings, groats), and boiled pasta. Vegetable and cereal soups are served uncooked, beetroots, borscht, and cabbage soup vegetarian, dairy, fruit soups are allowed. To improve the taste of dishes, various sauces and spices can be used. As for drinks, not only tea and rosehip broth can be taken but also coffee with milk, vitamin teas, non-acidic fruit, and vegetable juices.

Black coffee, cocoa, cold and carbonated drinks remain contraindicated.

Of the greatest importance in the prevention of exacerbations of chronic pancreatitis are abstinence from alcoholic beverages and smoking.

Patients in remission are prescribed low- and medium-mineralized mineral waters containing bicarbonates, sulfate ion, and divalent sulfur. Mineral waters are taken in a warm form (37–40 °C) with a course of up to 3-4 weeks. The dosage of mineral waters is strictly individual.

In hospitals, patients are recommended food that meets the requirements of a standard well-balanced diet, which provides the necessary biochemical, mechanical, and thermal sparing of the digestive system.

3.3 Chronic Pancreatitis with Incretory Insufficiency

A progressive pathological process with damage to the entire pancreas (including Langerhans cells) causes the development of not only excretory but also incretory insufficiency. This condition leads to the development of insulin and glucagon deficiency and the development of secondary diabetes mellitus.

The diet of patients with advanced endocrine pancreatic insufficiency is based on the principles of nutrition for patients with diabetes mellitus with the changes necessary for chronic pancreatitis.

To develop an individual diet, they are most often taken as the basic diet N°5 while excluding foods and dishes containing a large amount of easily digestible carbohydrates. Semolina, rice, oatmeal, potatoes, confectionery, and flour products (white wheat bread), sugar, and sweets are excluded. Buckwheat is recommended for cereals. Allow special diabetic or gray wheat bread from wholemeal flour in a limited amount (not more than 250g/day). When cooking cutlets, it is recommended to introduce fresh cottage cheese instead of bread (per 100g of meat - 50g of cottage cheese). Various sweeteners are widely used. Compotes, jellies, mousses are prepared with the addition of saccharin or xylitol. Foods rich in carbohydrates are distributed evenly throughout the day, or their consumption is timed to the time of the appointment of antidiabetic drugs.

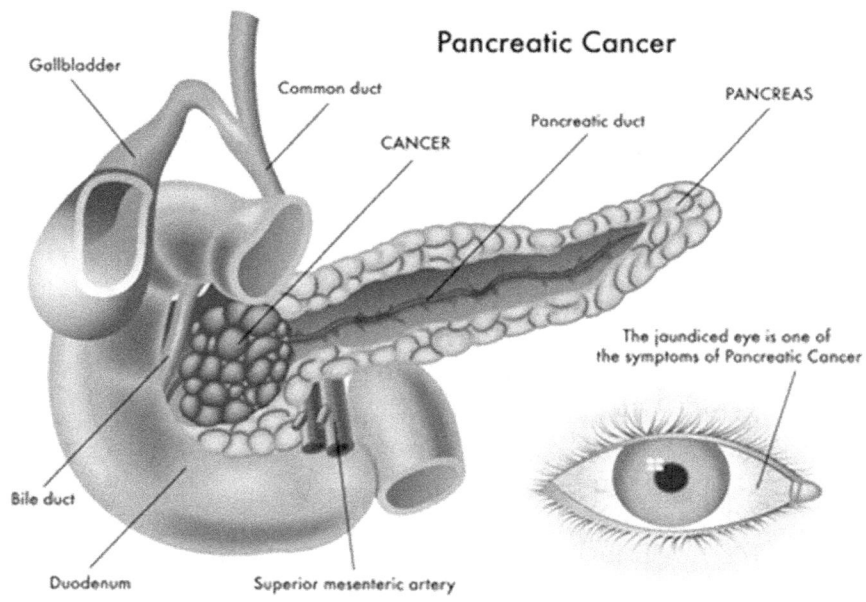

3.4 Sample Menus

3.4.1 Pancreatic Insufficiency

3.4.1.1 In the Period of Exacerbation of Chronic Pancreatitis;

- 1st breakfast: boiled tongue, carrot puree, and tea with milk.

- 2nd breakfast: steamed souffle from cottage cheese and baked apple.

- Lunch: vegetarian vegetable soup, boiled stroganoff from boiled meat, mashed potatoes, and fruit juice mousse.

- Snack: grated cheese, rosehip broth, crackers made of protein and wheat bread.

- Dinner: meatballs, fish, buckwheat milk porridge, tea, and diabetic cookies.

- At night: kefir.

- For the whole day: yesterday's protein-wheat bread of baking 200g, butter 20g.

3.4.1.2 In the Stage of Remission of Chronic Pancreatitis

- 1st breakfast: baked fish (low-fat species), stewed vegetables, tea, and cheese.

- 2-nd breakfast: steam omelet, rosehip broth, crackers made of protein, and wheat bread.

- Lunch: vegetable soup with meat broth, meatloaf, carrot puree, and fruit juice jelly.

- Snack: calcified cottage cheese, oatmeal jelly, crackers made of protein, and wheat bread.

- Dinner: carrot and pumpkin salad, stewed chicken, stewed vegetables in milk, and diabetic sausage.

- At night: kefir.

- For the whole day: yesterday's protein-wheat bread of baking 200g, butter 40g.

CLINICAL NUTRITION FOR BOWEL DISEASES

The diet of patients with intestinal pathology is given great attention. The intestine is the human body that performs one of the key roles in the digestion process. The intestine is divided into the small intestine and colon.

In the small intestine, through the cavity and parietal membrane digestion, hydrolysis of the main nutrients occurs, followed by absorption. Food proteins are cleaved by the action of enterokinase-activated pancreatic proteases to oligopeptides, which, in turn, are hydrolyzed by intestinal peptidases to form amino acids that undergo further absorption. Food triglycerides emulsified in the cavity of the small intestine are exposed to pancreatic lipase and are split into mono- and diglycerides, which are hydrolyzed inside the intestinal cells, turning into chylomicrons and transported to lymph. Carbohydrates received with food under the influence of pancreatic amylase break down to oligosaccharides in the small intestine cavity with further conversion under the action of intestinal disaccharidases into monosaccharides.

The colon serves as a reservoir for feces, plays an important role in the absorption of fluids, substances that are not absorbed in the small intestine, as well as in residual digestion.

Diet therapy recommended for intestinal diseases depends on the nature of the pathological process, the state of intestinal motor function, the presence or absence of food intolerance phenomena, the patient's age and gender, concomitant diseases, and individual taste preferences of the patient.

4.1 Basics of Clinical Nutrition for Intestinal Disorders
4.1.1 Objectives

With the help of a properly designed diet, the following clinical problems are solved:

- Normalization of intestinal motor activity

- Prevention of food intolerance

- Replenishment of the deficiency of essential nutrients

- Normalization of the composition of intestinal microflora in dysbiotic disorders

4.1.2 Principles

The basic principles of clinical nutrition are unchanged for all diseases of the intestine.

- Clinical nutrition should contribute to a targeted effect on metabolism; it should both heal and prevent the exacerbation of diseases.

- It is necessary to observe the correct diet: eat regularly at the same hours.

- It is necessary to diversify the diet.

- Clinical nutrition should be individualized: not a disease is treated, but a patient.

- The balance of the diet: it is necessary to take into account the calorie content and composition of the main products.

- Proper cooking is needed.

- When compiling an individual diet, it is imperative to take into account concomitant diseases.

- Clinical nutrition most effectively contributes to recovery if it is used in combination with other therapeutic factors: lifestyle changes, physical activation, the use of mineral waters, etc.

4.1.3 Classification of foods and dishes according to their effect on intestinal motility

When preparing a diet for patients with intestinal diseases, it is necessary to take into account the effect of foods and dishes on intestinal motility. All products are divided into three groups:

1. Products that enhance intestinal motility - brown bread, raw vegetables and fruits, dried fruits, especially prunes, dried apricots and apricots, bread containing bran, legumes, oatmeal, buckwheat and barley groats (compared to semolina and rice), sinewy meat, pickles, marinades, canned snacks, smoked meats, carbonated drinks, beer, kvass, fatty foods, very sweet dishes, especially in combination with organic acids, sour-milk drinks, koumiss, sour varieties of berries and fruits, and cold food.

2. Products that weaken intestinal motility - products rich in tannin (blueberries, bird cherry, strong tea, cocoa), viscous substances (mucous soups, mashed cereals, jelly), warm and hot dishes.

3. Indifferent products - steam dishes from low-fat and non-fatty varieties of meat and poultry (soufflé, dumplings, meatballs), boiled low-fat fish, wheat bread from premium flour stale or in the form of crackers, freshly made fresh cottage cheese.

4.2 Diarrhea Syndrome

One of the most common clinical symptoms in bowel disease is diarrhea.

Diarrhea is understood as frequent (as a rule, more than 2-3 times a day) bowel movement with the release of liquid and gruel-like bowel movements. The water content in feces with diarrhea increases to 85–95% and the mass of feces is more than 200g/day. Sometimes with diarrhea, the frequency of the stool does not exceed 1-2 times a day, but the feces have a more liquid consistency than normal. The acute diarrhea syndrome observed in acute intestinal infections is commonly referred to in cases where its duration does not exceed 2-3 weeks.

Diarrhea can develop in many diseases of the small and large intestine: acute intestinal infections, irritable bowel syndrome, celiac disease, and other fermentopathies, Crohn's disease, ulcerative colitis, carcinoid syndrome, and cancer of various intestines.

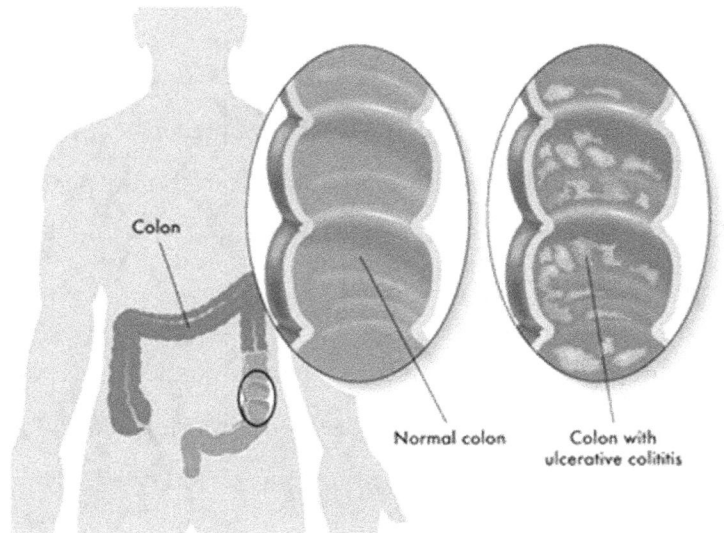

4.2.1 Principles

- The diet is aimed at reducing intestinal motor activity.

- It is necessary to limit the diet of mechanical and chemical irritants of the gastrointestinal tract.

- It is necessary to exclude products that enhance fermentation and putrefactive processes in the intestine.

- It is necessary to exclude products rich in essential oils (turnip, radish, sorrel, spinach, onions, garlic, and mushrooms).

- The temperature of food and drinks is at least 15-60 °C (i.e. only in the form of heat).

- The use of tannin-rich foods in the diet is recommended.

- It is recommended that foods containing simple carbohydrates be included in the diet.

4.2.2 Stages

- In the case of profuse severe diarrhea and severe dyspeptic symptoms, 1-2 "hungry" days are first prescribed, during which the patient is allowed to take 1.5–2 L of liquid per day in the form of strong tea with lemon and sugar 5–6 times a day (or rosehip decoction).

- In the future, the patient is recommended diet N°4 or diet N°4a. These diets are physiologically inferior and monotonous; therefore, they are prescribed for only 2–5 days.

- Then, as the severity of diarrhea, dyspeptic, and pain syndromes decreases, the patients are transferred to a physiologically complete diet N°4b for a period of 1-2 months to several years until the stool is completely normalized.

- In the phase of remission (after complete normalization of the stool), patients are prescribed diet N°4c, expanding the diet by eating the same dishes as in diet N°4b, but not in pureed form. Diet N°4c allows to restore the disturbed functions of the digestive system.

- The transfer from one diet to another is carried out by the zigzag method, that is, against the background of diet N°4b 1-2 times a week, diet N°4c is prescribed. With good tolerance of the diet, the patient is completely transferred to a new diet.

- After diet N°4c, a well-balanced diet can be assigned.

4.3 Intestinal Dyspepsia

Distinguish between fermentative and putrefactive intestinal dyspepsia. If a patient has dyspepsia, the necessary adjustments are introduced into the diet, depending on the type of dyspepsia.

4.3.1 Fermentative Dyspepsia

Fermentative dyspepsia is characterized by painful increased gas formation in the intestines (flatulence, rumbling in the stomach). There is a loss of appetite, pain in the abdominal cavity, and rapid fatigue. Typically, abundant gas is discharged. Gases are usually not offensive. Moderate diarrhea. Feces are usually light without any admixture of mucus and blood. Feces have an acid reaction.

Fermentative dyspepsia is usually caused by the predominance of sick food in the diet with an excess of easily digestible carbohydrates, which stimulate the suppression of normal intestinal flora and promote the growth of conditionally pathogenic aerobic microorganisms. At the same time, fermentation of sugars develops with the formation of large quantities of water and gases, as well as acetic and butyric acids, leading to a decrease in intestinal ph.

To reduce the fermentation processes in the daily diet of patients, it is necessary to reduce the amount of carbohydrates to 200–250g, and in severe cases, to 150g. The easily digestible, rapidly absorbed carbohydrates, which are rich in white cereals, mashed potatoes, jelly, sweet fruits and dried fruits, sweets (honey, jam, sweets, butter biscuits, etc.), white wheat bread, and muffin.

To reduce the transit rate of intestinal contents, the intake of dietary fiber contained in baked goods from whole ground grain with bran, nuts, legumes, dried fruits, cabbage, raw vegetables, and fruits is limited.

In patients with flatulence, products that stimulate gas formation are excluded or sharply limited (sweet varieties of apples, bananas, grapes, legumes, cabbage varieties - white cabbage, broccoli, Brussels sprouts, colored, whole milk, turnip, cucumbers, oats, carbonated drinks, etc.). Also, foods rich in essential oils (turnips, radishes, radishes, sorrel, spinach, onions, garlic, and mushrooms) are excluded.

The daily amount of protein, on the contrary, should be increased to 120-130g by prescribing boiled meat and fish of low-fat varieties, buckwheat, and oatmeal, protein omelets, and soy isolates.

Decoctions and infusions of medicinal plants are introduced into the diet of patients, suppressing fermentation processes (mint, chamomile, lingonberry, barberry, dogwood, dogrose, raspberry, strawberry, calendula, sage, etc.). Herbs are administered carefully, starting from 50ml/day, then, subject to good tolerance, increase to 200ml/day. The daily dose is divided into 3-4 doses.

When cooking, spices can be used (bay leaf, cloves, red and black pepper).

4.3.2 Putrid Dyspepsia

Putrid dyspepsia is characterized by intoxication (headache and weakness). Spasms and pains develop in the distal rectum. Flatulence with putrefactive dyspepsia is not as pronounced as with fermentation. The gas discharge is less, but the gases are more offensive. The stool is usually liquid or mushy, brown, with a sharp putrid smell, and contains pieces of undigested food.

Putrefactive dyspepsia develops as a result of prolonged eating mainly of products containing a large amount of protein, which leads to excessive growth of conditionally pathogenic anaerobes and pathogenic microbes that cause putrefactive processes in the intestine with the formation of toxic metabolic products. Methane, methyl mercaptan, hydrogen sulfide, indole, and skatol are formed in the intestines, which irritate the intestinal mucosa and cause frequent stools.

For the first 1-2 days, a patient with putrefactive dyspepsia is recommended hunger. A rosehip broth and slightly sweet tea can be drunk.

After 2 days, simple carbohydrates are prescribed - sweets, crackers, from the 5th day - rice porridge cooked in milk diluted half with water. Vegetable dishes, fermented milk products (yogurts, sour cream, fermented baked milk, acidophilus, kefir), which are used in 100–150ml 2–4 times a day, are shown.

With putrefactive dyspepsia in the diet, it is necessary to limit proteins to 30-50g/day. The consumption of protein foods is reduced - meat, fish, cheese, cottage cheese, legumes, nuts, eggs, semolina, buckwheat, and oatmeal.

The daily quota of fats is also reduced to 25-30g/day.

The amount of carbohydrates, on the contrary, is increased to 400-450g/day.

Increase dietary fiber intake. Cooked, stewed, and raw vegetables are sequentially introduced into the diet of a patient with dietary fiber. The appointment of vegetarian days is shown.

The growth of the anaerobic flora is suppressed by apricot, blackcurrant, mountain ash, cranberries, caraway seeds, infusions and decoctions of lemon balm, wormwood, pomegranate, oak bark, galanga, alder cones, oak leaves, thyme, sage, plantain, dandelion, and Icelandic moss.

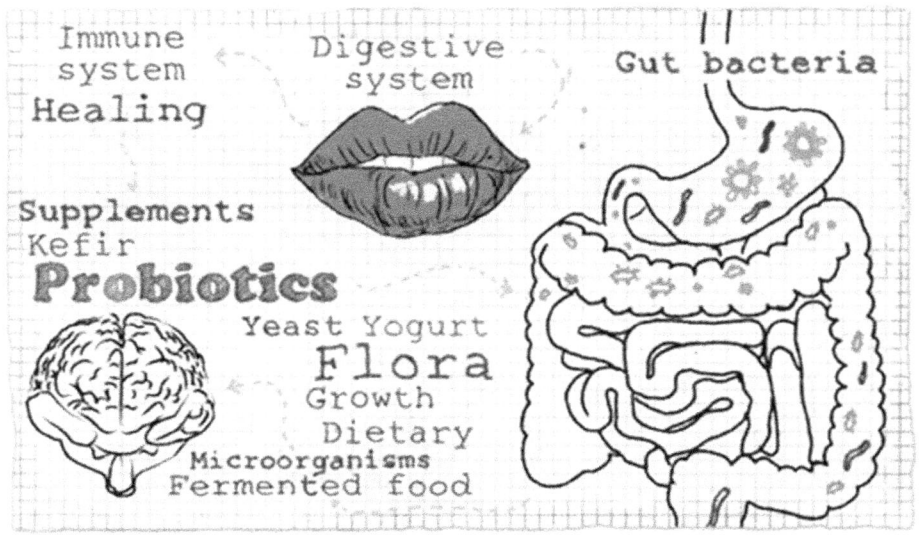

4.4 Diseases of the Intestine with Diarrhea

- In the presence of carcinoid tumors of the intestine, diet N°4 is recommended, but with high protein content and with a restriction of foods containing a lot of serotonin (walnuts, pineapples, kiwi, plums, tomatoes, eggplant, bananas, etc.) and its predecessor, 5-oxytryptophan (meat). Abundant meat food in patients with carcinoids can provoke a flushing syndrome (redness of the skin, dizziness, nausea, vomiting, diarrhea, shortness of breath, tachycardia, and change in blood pressure).

- With ischemic colitis, foods causing flatulence are excluded from the diet of patients. In order to reduce the spasm of the mesenteric vessels after eating, patients are recommended to lie for 2-3 hours with a warm heating pad on their stomachs.

- In chronic inflammatory bowel diseases (Crohn's disease, ulcerative colitis), Whipple's disease, patients are recommended to increase the daily protein quota to 1.5–2g/kg body weight. It is important to exclude dietary fiber from the diet. In some cases, in severe diseases, artificial nutrition is carried out - enteral and parental nutrition.

- In the case of amyloidosis of the small intestine, the intake of foods rich in casein (milk, cheese) is limited. It is recommended to increase products containing starch (potatoes, rice, and corn).

- With a number of diseases, diarrhea is one of the clinical manifestations of malabsorption syndrome. In this case, the development of protein-energy deficiency, lipid metabolism disorders, and multivitamin deficiency is possible. Mineral metabolism also suffers, as absorption of calcium, phosphorus, sodium, potassium, and iron decreases. A significant role in the treatment of malabsorption syndrome is given to clinical nutrition. Patients are prescribed a physiologically complete diet with high protein content, normal carbohydrate content and a moderate amount of fat, in which triglycerides containing fatty acids with a short or medium carbon chain length are introduced. In the case of malabsorption syndrome, the amount of proteins is increased to 130–135g by prescribing protein-rich products (low-fat varieties of meat and fish, dairy products, and egg white). Adequate intake of protein from the food stimulates anabolic processes, activates enzyme systems and increases the body's defenses. Sometimes the diet is supplemented by the inclusion of dietary products with specially defined properties that contribute not only to the compensation of losses of nutrients but also to the creation of optimal conditions for intestinal function. They can be used not only as a supplement to the main diet but also as a full daily diet. Parenteral nutrition is widely used to treat severe malabsorption syndrome, but also creating optimal conditions for intestinal function. Moreover, in recent years, they are the more often prescribed combined nutrition (parenteral and enteral nutrition). Along with daily infusions of amino acid mixtures, fat emulsions, and glucose solutions, nourishing substrates are introduced through a nasogastric tube in a droplet way (at a speed of 40-60 cap/min) or in sips through a tube gradually carry out the transition to normal oral nutrition.

4.5 Constipation Syndrome

The term "constipation" means persistent and prolonged dysfunction of the colon with a decrease in stool frequency less than 3 times a week with forced straining, occupying more than 25% of the time of the bowel movement.

By origin, constipation can be organic (colon cancer, Hirschsprung's disease, etc.) and functional (irritable bowel syndrome).

If there is a symptom of constipation, it is necessary to conduct a clinical examination of the patient, identify the cause of constipation and treat the underlying disease that caused constipation.

However, some measures can help normalize or improve intestinal motility (especially if there is a symptom of functional constipation).

When compiling a diet for a patient with constipation, preference is given to products that enhance intestinal motility, as well as rich in dietary fiber. Dietary fibers (non-digestible carbohydrates, fiber, and ballast substances) are substances of various chemical nature (alcohols, polysaccharides) that do not break down in the small intestine but undergo bacterial fermentation in the colon.

Highly soluble dietary fiber (which absorbs water and forms a gel, lowers cholesterol, blood sugar, for example, pectin, gums) and little or insoluble dietary fiber (which pass through the gastrointestinal tract almost unchanged, adsorb large amounts of water, affect motility intestines, for example - cellulose, hemicellulose, lignin).

According to WHO recommendations, 25–35g of ballast substances per day is considered to be the accepted norm in the body with food eaten. To comply with these standards, the WHO recommends a daily intake of at least 400g of fresh vegetables and fruits.

A decrease in fiber diet increases the risk of colon cancer, irritable bowel syndrome, constipation, diverticulosis of the intestine, hiatal hernia, cholelithiasis, diabetes mellitus, coronary heart disease, obesity, varicose veins, and venous thrombosis.

Enrichment of the diet with fiber, necessary for patients suffering from constipation, is carried out, including in the diet vegetables, fruits, dried fruits, and cereals, rich in ballast substances or special concentrates of dietary fiber.

According to the content of dietary fiber, food products vary significantly. Products rich in ballast substances include baked goods made from whole ground grain or containing a significant amount of bran, undesirable biscuits; buckwheat, barley, oatmeal, nuts (almonds, peanuts, pistachios), legumes, cabbage, apricots, blackberries, coconut, dried fruits, kiwi, parsley, popcorn, beets, carrots, and seaweed.

A patient suffering from constipation, in the absence of contraindications, is usually prescribed diet N°3 and in hospitals a standard diet.

For patients suffering from constipation, the use of a variety of biologically active micronutrients, including various dietary fibers, is recommended.

The most common is the use of wheat bran - a natural product containing vitamins and minerals (in their absence, oatmeal can be used). 100g of wheat bran contains 17g of protein, 4g of fat, 53g of fiber, 12g of starch, and 6g of minerals. Before use, bran must be poured with boiling water for 15 minutes so that they swell and become softer, then drain the supernatant. Swollen bran is added to compotes, cereals, jelly, meatballs, soups and other dishes or consumed in its pure form. Usually, start with 1 teaspoon 3 times a day, gradually increasing to 1-2 tablespoons 3 times a day (the dose is increased every 3-4 days for 2-4 weeks). When a laxative effect is achieved, reduce the dose to 1.5–2 teaspoons 3 times a day, on average, treatment is continued for at least 6 weeks.

In patients with constipation, the intake of bran causes an increase in the mass of feces, water content in them, a decrease in the time for the contents to move through the intestines, and frequent stools. At first, bloating may increase, and a feeling of fullness may occur, but these phenomena are transient. Coarse bran more effectively reduces intracavitary pressure and accelerate the transit of intestinal contents.

However, it should be remembered that with prolonged and excessive consumption of dietary fiber, there is a 1.5–2% decrease in the absorption of vitamins, macro- and microelements (calcium, phosphorus, magnesium, iron, zinc), therefore, normally their quantity should not exceed 25–35g/day, therapeutic dose - 40g/day, the maximum dose is 60g/day.

Dietary fiber enhances gas production in patients with flatulence and pain in patients with severe intestinal motility, which should be considered when choosing a dose of bran and diet in such patients. In such cases, at first, a diet low in dietary fiber is used, except products that cause increased gas formation (legumes, cabbage, sorrel, and spinach).

To reduce and subsequently eliminate intestinal cramps, antispastic drugs are prescribed, then foods containing fiber of delicate, and subsequently rougher consistency are gradually added to food. In addition to dietary fiber, products containing organic acids are indicated to speed up bowel movement. Such products include sour milk, koumiss, fresh kefir, acidophilus, yogurt, sour fruits, dried fruits (figs, dried apricots, dates), fruit and vegetable juices. Moreover, juices, in comparison with fruits, sometimes have a more pronounced laxative effect, since the concentration of sugars and organic acids in juices is higher, especially in plum and peach.

With functional constipation, the patient's diet includes sugary substances (honey, syrup, sugar, marmalade, marshmallow, marshmallows, iris, milk and cream caramels, preserves and jams from sweet varieties of berries and fruits).

The permissible amount of sodium chloride is 12–15g/day. Therefore, dishes rich in sodium chloride (pickles, marinades, and herring) are recommended to stimulate the motor activity of the intestine.

Caffeinated drinks, white grape wines, cold dishes, products containing fructose, sorbitol as sweeteners are allowed for the same purpose.

The intake of mineral waters is recommended for constipation with increased contractile activity of the intestine, with the presence of spastic pain in the abdomen, as well as "sheep" feces. In the case of intestinal hypomotility, when the intestinal motor activity is reduced, as evidenced by volumetric feces, the high mineralized water is recommended. Cold mineral water is taken on an empty stomach 1–1.5 cups 2-3 times a day on an empty stomach 1–1½ hours before meals in a few weeks. Such courses are repeated several times a year. For constipation with increased contractile activity of the intestine, for pain in the abdomen, it is preferable to take warm mineral water.

If there are no special contraindications (heart disease, swelling), a patient suffering from constipation should drink about 1.5–2 liters of fluid per day. With functional constipation, the use of the correct diet with sufficient patient allows in most cases to eliminate constipation or, in any case, reduce it without prescribing laxatives.

4.6 Excessive Gas Formation in the Intestine

Many patients complain of painful bloating, rumbling, and transfusion in the abdomen. At the same time, patients do not always have bowel movements (diarrhea or constipation).

To reduce the phenomena of flatulence, foods and drinks containing a large amount of gases (carbonated drinks, whipped cream, soufflé; drinks prepared using a mixer) should be excluded from the diet of patients.

It is advisable to limit products that stimulate the processes of gas formation in the intestine: dishes with high-fat content, whole milk, legumes, broccoli; white cabbage, asparagus, and cauliflower, nuts, sweet apples, melons, bananas, wheat sprouts, pasta, potatoes, artichokes, yeast, honey, cane sugar, sugar from sugar beets, mustard, and leeks.

4.7 Diverticular Bowel Disease

Diverticular bowel disease is a disease characterized by the formation of diverticula of the intestinal wall. Diverticular disease is widespread in developed countries. Several factors obviously play a role in its formation: weakness of the intestinal wall, impaired intestinal motor activity, and increased intracavitary pressure.

It is generally recognized that in the prevention and treatment of diverticular disease, food rich in dietary fiber plays a crucial role.

4.7.1 Principles

- The diet should contain a large amount of plant fiber - dietary fiber. It is advisable to add bran (gradually over a period of 2-4 weeks from 5-10 to 20g/day).

- The introduction of a sufficient amount of bran into food allows to increase the amount of feces, reduce their transit time and, accordingly, reduce intracavitary pressure.

- Other caloformants (e.g., lactulose) do not have such a positive effect on intracavitary pressure.

- It is necessary to exclude food containing small, poorly and indigestible components: fruits with small seeds (kiwi, grapes seeds). When stuck in the cavity of the diverticulum, they can cause diverticulitis.

- Particular care should be taken to thoroughly cleanse the fish of small bones, which can lead to perforation of the diverticulum.

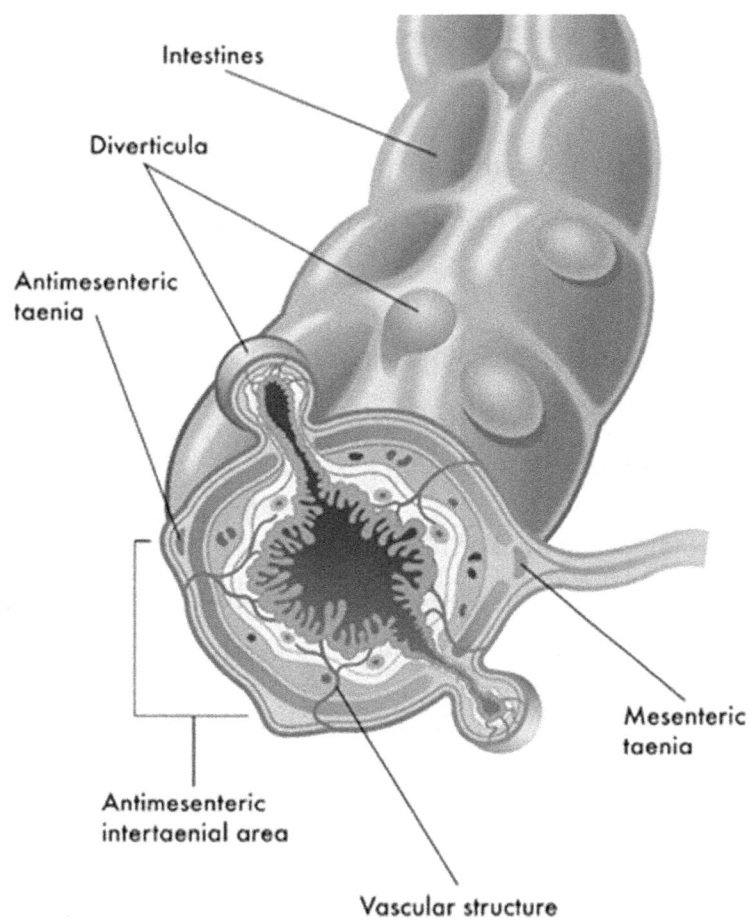

4.8 Fermentopathies (enzyme deficiency enteropathies)

In recent decades, much attention has been paid to the study of a group of diseases called "enzyme deficiency enteropathy" or enzymeopathy. In patients with these diseases, a decrease in the activity of key digestive tract enzymes occurs. As a result of this, digestion and absorption of food ingredients are disrupted, and malabsorption syndrome develops.

Distinguish between congenital (primary) and acquired (secondary) enzyme deficiency enteropathy.

The most famous example of primary fermentopathy is celiac disease or celiac enteropathy.

Secondary enzyme deficiency enteropathies develop against the background of inflammatory or degenerative changes in the mucous membrane of the small intestine.

4.8.1 Celiac Disease

Celiac disease (celiac enteropathy) is a chronic autoimmune disease caused by impaired gluten tolerance, which results in inflammation of the mucous membrane of the small intestine and malabsorption syndrome.

The main treatment for celiac disease is a lifelong diet, the main principle of which should be the exclusion of all products containing gluten.

Such products include all products, including barley, millet, wheat, rye, and oats. This group includes the specified cereals, white and black bread, pasta, dumplings, pancakes, cakes, pastries, cookies, gingerbread cookies, ice cream, and puddings. Grains intolerable to patients with celiac disease are found in some alcoholic beverages (beer, whiskey), in instant soups, instant coffee drinks. Flour can be added to yogurts, glazed curds, sausages, cheeses, canned goods, ketchup, and sauces.

For patients with celiac disease, a special gluten-free diet (N°4d) is developed.

In the diet, they observe the principle of mechanical and biochemical sparing of the gastrointestinal tract, exclude foods and dishes that increase fermentation processes. Limit substances that stimulate the secretion of the stomach, pancreas, and products that adversely affect the functional state of the liver. Depending on the functional state of the intestine, food is given in pureed form (during periods of diarrhea) or without special grinding (with normalization of the stool).

Dietary restrictions must be strictly met by the patient since even 100mg of gluten-containing foods (a few crumbs of bread) can cause atrophy of the villi of the small intestine. Products with a gluten content of more than 1mg/100g of product are considered unacceptable for patients with celiac disease.

On the contrary, with perfect adherence to the gluten-free diet in most patients, restoration of the structure and function of intestinal villi occurs within 3–6 months.

Typically, diet N°4d is supplemented by the exclusion of lactose and allergens. Children of the 1st year of life can be prescribed soy mixtures or mixtures based on casein hydrolyzate.

Gluten-free cereals and vegetables (rice, corn, and legumes) are allowed. In the preparation of various dishes (pastries, sauces), rice, and cornflour, potato starch is used as substitutes for wheat flour. Buckwheat porridge is indicated in limited quantities.

4.8.2 Disaccharidase Deficiency

Disaccharidase deficiency is a violation of the digestion and absorption of disaccharides (lactose, sucrose, trehalose, maltose, and isomaltose), due to a deficiency of the corresponding intestinal enzymes (lactase, sucrase, trehalase, maltase or isomaltase).

The clinical manifestations of various types of disaccharidase deficiency are identical, and the only difference is in what foods cause an exacerbation of the disease.

Intestinal disaccharidases break down food disaccharides into monosaccharides that are absorbed into the blood. Violation of membrane hydrolysis leads to the formation in the intestinal cavity of a large amount of undissolved to the end and non-adsorbed substances that contribute to an increase in osmotic pressure in the intestinal lumen. Increased osmotic pressure, in turn, increases the secretion of fluid and motor activity of the intestine, causing the appearance of the main clinical symptom of all fermentopathies - diarrhea.

Significant in these diseases is the fact that the appearance of clinical symptoms (exacerbation of the disease) is caused only by the use of foods containing those carbohydrates, the hydrolysis of which is difficult due to the deficiency of a certain type of disaccharidase.

The severity of the clinical manifestations of fermentopathy and the severity of malabsorption depend on the degree of deficiency of the enzyme and the content of carbohydrates hydrolyzed by it in the taken food product.

4.8.3 Lactase Deficiency

Lactase deficiency is the most common variant of disaccharide deficiency.

Congenital or acquired lactase deficiency is manifested only when eating milk and dairy products containing lactose (milk sugar).

There is a congenital lack of lactase production (alactasia), as well as primary and secondary lactase deficiency.

The main treatment for patients with absolute lactase deficiency (alactasia) is a complete rejection of milk and dairy products.

In patients with primary or secondary lactase deficiency, restriction of milk and dairy products is required. Moreover, the degree of restriction should be strictly individual, since some patients cannot tolerate only milk, but can eat fermented milk products with a low content of lactose. And patients with an insignificant degree of hypolactasia without harm to health can consume even small amounts of fresh milk (up to 100-150 ml per day). In such cases, milk is allowed to be taken on an empty stomach, slowly, in small portions, no more than 1-2 times a week.

When lactose deficiency is detected in infants, they are transferred to food with special low-lactose or lactose-free mixtures, in which, with the help of different types of processing (chemical casein precipitation, spray drying), the lactose level is reduced to almost zero. Lactose-free mixtures on packages are labeled "SL" (sine lactose) or "LF" (lactose-free). Lactose-free soy-based mixtures can be used.

4.8.3.1 Classification of Low-Lactose Foods

A low-lactose mixture is a powder that resembles milk powder in appearance and taste.

The composition of such mixtures also includes corn oil and milk fats in a ratio of 25:75, sucrose, malt extract or dextrin-maltose, starch, flour for baby and diet food, vitamins A, D, E, PP, C, group B, macro - and trace elements (iron, sodium, potassium, calcium, phosphorus, and magnesium).

Low-lactose foods come in several forms;

- Low-lactose milk mixture with malt extract (for children up to 2 months).

- Low-lactose milk mixture with flour (rice, buckwheat, oatmeal) and oat flour for children older than 2 months.

- Low-lactose milk for children older than 6 months and as a substitute for milk for cooking.

- Low-lactose egg-based mixture with sugar, margarine, and rice flour.

- In dairy kitchens, there is special lactose-free milk, on which cereals for children can be prepared.

Foods always high in milk sugar;

- Milk powder
- Whole milk
- Skimmed milk
- Whey and all products based on it

Products that almost always contain some amounts of milk sugar – 'hidden lactose;'

- Milk and dairy products
- Sausages in packaging, including boiled ham
- Soups in bags
- Ready-made sauces
- Bakery products
- Nut butter
- Icecream
- Breadcrumbs
- Cakes and pies
- Dumplings
- Croquettes with cheese
- Hamburgers

- Cheeseburgers
- Ham
- Ketchup
- Mustard
- Mayonnaise
- Amplifiers of taste
- Astringent for sauces
- Sweeteners in finished packaged products
- Condensed milk
- Loosespices, broths
- Chocolate bars, sweets such as candy, chocolate (except for some varieties of dark chocolate)
- Cocoa Powder
- Nutritional supplements
- Light sauces
- Puddings, mashed soups
- Donuts and omelets
- Mashed potatoes
- Saccharin tablets

Lactose-Free Products;

- Fruit
- Vegetables
- Jam
- Honey
- Coffee
- Tea
- Vegetable oil
- Fruit juices
- Figs
- Vermicelli
- Soy milk and soy drinks
- Raw meat
- Raw fish
- Poultry meat
- Chicken egg
- Any kind of sugar, except milk (sorbitol, fructose)
- Liquid saccharin

- Potatoes
- Legumes
- Corn
- Syrups
- Vegetable juices
- Salt
- Nuts
- Alcoholic drinks

Lactose content in some foods;

In grams per 100g of product:

- Dessert cream - 2.8-6.3
- Coffee whitener - 10.0
- Powderedmilkyogurt - 4.7
- Wholemilkyogurt (3.5%) - 4.0
- Milk yogurt (1.5%) - 4.1
- Milk yogurt (3.5%) - 4.0
- Natural yogurt - 3.2

- Creamy yogurt - 3.7
- Fruit nonfat yogurt - 3.1
- Fat-free fruit yogurt - 3.0
- Creamy fruit yogurt - 3.2
- Yogurticecream - 6.9
- Cocoa - 4.6
- Mashed potatoes - 4.0
- Semolina porridge - 6.3
- Rice porridge in milk - 18.0
- Kefir - 6.0
- Low-fat kefir - 4.1
- Sausages - 1.0-4.0
- Margarine - 0.1
- Butter - 0.6
- Sour milk - 5.3
- Nonfat milk - 4.9
- Pasteurizedmilk (3.5%) - 4.8
- Condensed milk (7.5%) - 9.2

- Condensed milk (10%) - 12.5
- Condensed milk with sugar - 10.2
- Powdered milk - 51.5
- Skimmed milk powder - 52.0
- Wholemilk (3.5%) - 4.8
- Whole milk powder - 38.0
- Milkshakes - 5.4
- Milk chocolate - 9.5
- Icecream - 6.7
- Milk ice cream - 1.9-7.0
- Icecreamicecream - 1.9
- Creamy icecream - 5.1-6.9
- Fruit icecream - 5.1-6.9
- Nougat - 25.0
- Buttermilk - 3.5
- Dry buttermilk - 44.2
- Donuts - 4.5
- Pudding - 2.8-6.3

- Whippedcream (10%) - 4.8
- Whipped cream (30%) - 3.3
- Coffee cream - 3.8
- Pasteurizedcream - 3.3
- Wholepasteurizedcream - 3.1
- Sour cream (10%) - 2.5
- Dry whey - 70.0
- Gouda cheese (45%) - 2.0
- Camembert cheese (45%) - 0.1-1.8
- Mozzarella cheese - 0.1-3.1
- Parmesan cheese - 0.05-3.2
- Roquefort cheese - 2.0
- Cottage cheese (20%) - 2.7
- Cottage cheese (40%) - 2.6
- Fat-free cottage cheese - 3.2

Products approved for use with lactase deficiency;

- Products with components such as milk protein and acid, modified starch, astringents and thickeners, flavorings, and spices do not contain milk sugar.

- Low lactose infant formula.

- Meat, poultry, fish.

- The eggs.

- Vegetable oil.

- Lard.

- All fruits and vegetables.

- Natural flour, bread.

- Regular sugar, glucose, fructose.

- It is recommended to include vegetables (broccoli, cabbage, and turnips), fish (sardines, salmon), soy products, eggs, and liver in the diet. These foods are a source of vitamin D, which is essential for the absorption of calcium.

- Cheeses are divided by maturity: the longer the cheese ripens, the less milk sugar remains in it. Thus, hard and semi-solid varieties lose most of their lactose.

- Fatty and bold creams contain less lactose than milk; therefore, in exceptional cases and small amounts, their use is allowed.

- Butter contains very little lactose and is also used in small quantities; therefore, there can be no doubt about its digestibility. The higher the fat content in the product, the less lactose it contains.

- Bakery products, pies, waffles, cookies usually contain milk sugar and, therefore, their use is not advisable.

- An alternative to cow's milk can be soy milk, which is a plant product; it is soy puree that has been heat-treated, and water. This product does not contain chemical additives; it is rich in proteins, and does not contain sugar and cholesterol. Perfect for preparing various dishes where the technology requires cow milk.

Products prohibited for use with lactase deficiency

If the list of ingredients of the consumed product contains lactose, milk sugar, milk powder, whole milk, skim milk, whey, whey products, then this product should be discarded.

- Cow milk, and all types of milk powder
- Cream with the addition of soy
- Liver, brains, pastes
- All kinds of sausages, ham

- Fresh cream, margarine
- Peas
- Beetroot
- Green beans
- Dried potatoes
- Lentils
- Factory-made milk drinks
- Sponge cake, pastries, bread with milk
- Productswithsoy
- Chocolate with milk, sweets with milk (toffee), caramel with milk
- Medicines in which milk sugar is added

4.8.4 Sucrose, Maltase and Isomaltase Deficiency

Distinguish between primary and secondary insufficiency of the production of these enzymes.

Sucrose and isomaltase deficiency is detected clinically when eating foods containing sucrose. Such patients should exclude from the food all products containing beet and cane sugar. They include all sweets, except honey.

Most fruits are allowed to be consumed, as well as products manufactured especially for patients with diabetes mellitus, with sweeteners (xylitol or sorbitol, saccharin).

Children with this type of fermentopathy in the first year of life are allowed to breast-feed with mother or donor (expressed) milk, as well as with cow's milk without added sugar. In this case, milk should not be diluted with decoctions, use flour and dextrin-maltose.

Starting from 3-4 months, little green vegetables, meat, eggs, fish, and ascorbic acid are introduced into the baby's diet.

Children who are on mixed or artificial feeding are given a mixture of cow's milk with glucose or fructose.

- A daily diet of a strict food for a child of 1.5 years with intolerance to sucrose and isomaltose.
- Breakfast: whole milk - 200g, glucose - 37g.
- Lunch: cauliflower - 200g, sunflower oil - 20g, greens - 5g, low-fat veal - 30g, lettuce - 20g, glucose - 25g.
- Snack: egg yolk - 1 piece, glucose - 20g, gelatin - 10g, water - 100ml.
- Dinner: lettuce - 100g, cottage cheese - 100g, glucose - 25g, dill tea - 100ml.
- Sucrose-free daily diet for a 2-year-old child with good tolerance to isomaltose.
- In the morning: cornbread - 10g, butter - 5g, liverwurst - 5g, whole milk - 150g, glucose - 20g.
- Lunch: lettuce - 100g, polished rice - 30g, low-fat mutton - 30g, greens - 5g, egg yolk - 1 piece, glucose - 25g.

- Snack: whole milk - 100ml, glucose - 25g, gelatin - 5g, 20% cream - 30ml.
- Dinner: whole milk - 200ml, glucose - 30g, cornbread - 10g, smoked sausage - 5g, butter - 5g.

Diet therapy is carried out under the constant supervision of a doctor and laboratory diagnostic methods.

If the condition improves, the diet can expand. However, some patients should follow a diet for life.

As a rule, recovery can occur by 10-12 years with a diet. In this case, at first, there is a good tolerance of starch, then sucrose.

4.8.5 Trehalase Deficiency

Signs of trehalase deficiency occur after eating mushrooms, which are the main source of trehalose. Patients with a deficiency of trehalose are shown to exclude mushrooms, mushroom sauces, and seasonings with the addition of mushrooms from food.

4.8.6 Monosaccharides Deficiency

The cause of food intolerance of some carbohydrates may be due to defects in the transport systems involved in the absorption of monosaccharides in the small intestine. In most cases, such defects are congenital and inherited. Very rarely, secondary acquired deficiency of absorption of monosaccharides develops.

Distinguish between glucose and galactose malabsorption syndrome, as well as fructose malabsorption syndrome.

Impaired absorption of these monosaccharides irritates the intestinal mucosa and increases the rate of transit of intestinal contents. Appearing diarrhea contributes to the loss of fluids, proteins, fats, vitamins, macro- and micronutrients.

4.8.6.1 Malabsorption Syndrome for Glucose and Galactose

The goal of clinical nutrition for glucose and galactose malabsorption syndrome is the exclusion of foods rich in glucose and galactose, which are almost all carbohydrates.

Treatment is carried out for 3 years with a special diet in which galactose is absent.

Treatment is carried out under the supervision of a pediatrician, nutritionist, optometrist, neuropathologist, under the supervision of a biochemical blood test for galactose.

The complexity of clinical nutrition lies in the fact that it is necessary to deprive a child of breast milk from the neonatal period, i.e., before the first symptoms of the disease appear.

At the slightest suspicion of intolerance, galactose and glucose of the newborn are transferred to food with special low-lactose or lactose-free mixtures, in which, with the help of various types of treatment (casein precipitation by chemical means, spray drying), the lactose level is reduced to almost zero. The low-lactose mixture with the malt extract is used in the first stages until the diagnosis is finally removed or made.

If the diagnosis was not confirmed during a biochemical blood test, then the baby again begins to receive breast milk.

The daily volume of milk mixtures, the frequency of feeding, and the timing of the introduction of complementary foods - all this is carried out according to the norms established for healthy children, except for offal, legumes, coffee, cocoa, and chocolate.

Children older than one year are allowed fruit sweets, marmalade, and jams. Fructose (100–300g/day) remains the only authorized source of carbohydrates for patients with this type of fermentopathy. Pears, figs, prunes, and grapes are high in fructose.

4.8.6.1.1 Principles

Early prescription of diet food (from the first feeding of the newborn, if there is a suspicion of this disease). If treatment is started from the first days of life, it is possible to prevent the development of cirrhosis, cataracts, and oligophrenia (dementia). If diet therapy is started at a later date, when the child already has a developmental delay and liver pathology, the disease can only be stopped without further deterioration. However, one can no longer count on recovery.

- Introduction to the diet of a full-fledged substitute for lactose-free female milk. Significant improvement can be achieved by eliminating milk and dairy products from the diet.

- Inclusion in the diet of the child as he grows a variety of permitted foods.

- Limit the use of milk and dairy products to pregnant women who are at high risk of having a baby with galactosemia. In cases where similar diseases in the family are known, milk is excluded from the pregnant woman's diet, as well as peas, beans, lentils, soybeans, young potatoes, cocoa, chocolate, liver, and other offal.

When monosaccharides deficiency is detected in infants, they are transferred to food with special low-lactose or lactose-free mixtures, in which, with the help of different types of treatment (chemically precipitated casein, spray drying), the lactose level is reduced to almost zero. Lactose-free mixtures on packages are labeled "LF" (lactose-free). Lactose-free soy-based mixtures can be used.

Menu using low-lactose milk for galactosemia (child's age – 7 months, weight – 8kg)

- First feeding. Low-lactose (12%) milk - 200ml.

- The second feeding. Porridge with low-lactose (12%) milk - 150ml, ghee - 5g, yolk - 1/2 pieces, bread - 50g, apple puree - 50g.

- Third feeding. Broth - 30ml, vegetable puree in low-lactose (12%) milk - 150g, vegetable oil - 5g, meat puree - 30g, bread - 5g, fruit jelly - 30ml.

- Fourth feeding. Low-lactose (12%) milk - 200ml, apple juice - 50ml, crackers - 5g.

- Fifth feeding. Low-lactose (12%) milk - 200ml.

4.8.6.2 Fructose Malabsorption Syndrome

With fructose malabsorption syndrome, eating fructose-rich foods is prohibited. The main sources of fructose are considered to be honey, sugarcane and beets, fruits, jams, carrots, cocoa, chicory, turnips.

Clinical nutrition consists of the exclusion from the diet of all products containing fructose in any form. Newborns are prescribed infant formula without sugar. Children of the first year receive milk formula containing only lactose and dextrin-maltose. Instead of fruit purees and juices, food is supplemented with glucose (from 30 to 60g). With the introduction of complementary foods earlier in healthy children, prescribe meat, fish, cheese, and eggs. Ascorbic acid is used without sugar.

As soon as fructose ceases to enter the body, appetite is restored, vomiting stops, and patients add to the mass.

Clinical nutrition is indicated for children up to 5-6 years old. Only after reaching this age, it is possible in limited quantities, under the supervision of a doctor and biochemical blood tests, to include products from the prohibited list in the child's nutrition.

Approved products for fructose malabsorption syndrome:

- Sick children are allowed female and cow milk. Powdered milk should be sugar-free (sucrose).

- All types of cheeses and natural dairy products (unsweetened) are allowed.

- Animal products are allowed, including meat, fish, and eggs.

- Fats are included in the diet with almost no restrictions (butter and vegetable oils).

- Lemons and chestnuts.

- From vegetables, green beans, watercress, lettuce, leek, cabbage, and spinach are allowed.

- The following products are also allowed: natural wheat or rye flour, rice, bread, semolina, tea, coffee, cocoa without sugar, glucose, maltose, dextrin-maltose, saccharin.

4.8.6.2.1 Prohibited Foods

It is forbidden to milk with the addition of sucrose, condensed milk, and sweetened sour-milk products.

- Sausages and canned food are excluded.

- All fruits are prohibited.

- Soy, flour with sucrose, biscuits, cakes, lemonade, and all carbonated fruit drinks, juices, syrups, sugar, jam, nougat, and sweets are prohibited.

- All medicines containing sugar, sorbitol (granules, dragees, powders, and pills) are prohibited.

CLINICAL NUTRITION AFTER OPERATIONS ON THE DIGESTIVE ORGANS

The most important factor in the postoperative rehabilitation of patients who underwent surgery of the digestive organs is clinical nutrition.

Diet therapy is aimed at meeting the plastic and energy needs of the patient's body. Proper nutrition helps reduce the incidence of complications and leads to a speedy recovery. The most important task of diet therapy in both inpatient and outpatient stages of metabolic rehabilitation is to overcome the protein, vitamin, mineral, and energy deficiencies that develop in most patients due to surgical trauma, fever, and malnutrition after surgery.

Surgery, regardless of the type of surgical intervention and the accompanying anesthesia, causes powerful metabolic changes in the body. The patient's body is affected by both specific factors of surgical trauma (blood and plasma loss, hypoxia, toxemia, impaired function of damaged organs), as well as non-specific factors, such as pain impulses, excitation of adrenergic and pituitary-adrenal systems.

Surgical stress is characterized by a sharp increase in the processes of catabolism, expressed metabolic disorders, especially protein and energy. The main causes of these disorders are the catabolic effect of adrenocorticotropic hormone and glucocorticoids, adrenaline and vasopressin, increased proteolysis in tissues, loss of protein from the wound that is separated from the wound, and increased energy expenditure with the utilization of our own proteins. At the same time, catabolism is not only enhanced, but protein synthesis is also inhibited. The destruction of glycogen in the liver and muscles (an easily accessible but small source of energy), triglycerides in adipose tissue, is considered part of the early neuroendocrine response to surgical trauma. Carbohydrate reserves in the body are limited, and therefore tissue proteins are actively involved in energy metabolism,

The duration and severity of the catabolic phase of stress during severe and extensive surgical interventions (resection and plastic surgery of the esophagus, stomach, and gastrectomy) hinder the long-term adaptation phase in the early postoperative period.

In patients undergoing surgery, in the immediate postoperative period, energy metabolism is sharply increased, mainly due to an inadequate increase in actual basal metabolism. Moreover, often the energy deficit reaches such values that even with the consumption of a normal diet (2500-3000kcal/day), patients still find themselves in conditions of severe protein-energy deficiency. In this case, there is a transition to complete or partial endogenous nutrition, which leads to a rapid (sometimes catastrophic) depletion of carbohydrate and fat reserves, as well as a significant loss of protein. These phenomena significantly worsen the course of regeneration processes, delay the progression of the postoperative wound process. There are prerequisites for the development of postoperative complications, including post-resection dystrophy.

There are two types of complications observed after operations on the digestive tract:

- Complications associated with the late onset of enteral nutrition, leading to gastro stasis, bloating, and insufficiency of anastomotic sutures.

- Infectious complications caused by a decrease in immune and nonspecific protection due to lack of nutrition, such as suppuration of a postoperative wound, congestive pneumonia, peritonitis, and sepsis.

5.1 After Surgery on the Esophagus

Diet therapy is an important part of the entire complex of postoperative rehabilitation of patients after surgery on the esophagus.

In the early stages after surgical treatment, the patient undergoes rehabilitation treatment in a surgical hospital, and then in the gastroenterological department, where the patient goes to aftercare. As a rule, 1.5-2 months after surgery are transferred to the outpatient treatment of the patient.

Clinical nutrition in the first months after surgery on the esophagus is carried out according to the principles of parenteral and enteral artificial nutrition.

By 4-6 months, the outpatient metabolic rehabilitation phase of patients is transferred to natural nutrition.

In prescribing a special diet designed for patients who underwent surgery on the esophagus, the following are obtainable:

The diet is physiologically complete, high in protein, with limited mechanical and chemical irritants of the mucous membrane of the esophagus.

After a four-month period after surgery, in the absence of complications, the diet should be expanded, a significant part of the dietary restrictions should be removed, and diet N°1 should be prescribed.

Subsequently, but not earlier than one year after the operation, subjects present a normalization of all functions of the gastrointestinal tract could progressively normalize their diet.

In those cases when patients undergo chemo or X-ray radiotherapy, a varied, complete food is justified for enhanced nutrition of high-calorie content, with a large number of high-grade proteins, fats, carbohydrates, and vitamins. These patients could be oriented to a high protein diet.

5.1.1 Basics of the diet therapy

A physiologically complete diet with a high protein content and normal fat content. The restriction of mechanical and chemical irritants of the mucous membrane of the esophagus, stomach, and the receptor apparatus of the gastrointestinal tract, the maximum restriction of nitrogenous extractives, refractory fats, and fat breakdown products are carried out. Strong stimulants of bile secretion and pancreatic secretion are excluded from the diet.

- The consumption of salt is limited.
- All dishes are steamed, mashed.
- The total amount of free fluid is 1.5 liters.
- Food temperature - hot dishes less than 50-60 °C; cold dishes over 15 °C.

5.1.1.1 Composition

Proteins 140g (of which 60% of animal origin), fats 110-115g, carbohydrates 400g, calories 2800-3000kcal, ascorbic acid 100mg, retinol 2mg, thiamine 4mg, riboflavin 4mg, nicotinic acid 30mg; calcium 0.8g, phosphorus not less than 1.6g, magnesium 0.5g, and iron 15mg.

- Salt is recommended to limit to 506g per day.

5.1.1.2 Recommended foods

- Bread products - yesterday's wheat bread, crackers made of wheat bread, cookies are not full, slightly sweet, and the bread is allowed no earlier than 1.5 months after the operation.

- Soups - on vegetable, cereal broths, mashed, excluding white cabbage and millet.

- Meat dishes - from lean beef, chicken, turkey, rabbit, veal (with removal of tendons) and dishes from low-fat fish - cod, pike perch, carp, pike, bream, saffron cod, silver hake, carp, ice, all in the form of mashed potatoes, souffle, meatballs, rolls, and cutlets.

- Egg and egg products - soft-boiled egg, not more than one egg per day, protein omelet.

- Milk and dairy products - milk with tea and other products or as part of various dishes, with tolerance - whole milk; kefir is included in 2.5-3 months after surgery; sour cream only as seasoning; freshly prepared non-acidic curd, mashed.

- Vegetables and greens - boiled, mashed vegetables; only cauliflower, boiled with butter, stewed squash and pumpkin, carrot, beetroot, and mashed potatoes.

- Fruits, berries, sweets - natural fruits and berries, fresh and dry in the form of unsweetened mashed compotes, jelly, mousses; baked apples, non-sour sugar-free varieties; fruits and berries with coarse fiber (pear, quince, persimmon) are not allowed; compotes, jelly on xylitol, while sugar, honey jam are limited.

- Cereals and pasta - unsweetened, mashed, viscous cereals, puddings, casseroles of rice, longitudinal cereals, oatmeal; pasta only finely chopped, boiled.

- Fats - butter, ghee, sunflower, refined; do not fry, but add to the dishes in kind.

- Snacks - cheese, mild grated, spawned caviar, a small amount of granular, jelly of boiled legs and boiled meat on gelatin (without extracts or additives).

- Sauces on vegetable broth, sour cream sauces, butter; flour for sauces excluding passer with butter.

- Drinks and juices - juices in the form of unsweetened fruit, berry, and vegetable; they should be diluted, only freshly prepared; decoctions of rose hips; weak tea, tea with milk, weak surrogate coffee on water and with milk.

5.1.1.3 Excluded Foods

- Products from butter and hot dough.

- Brains, liver, kidneys, lungs, meat, fish, mushroom soups, cabbage soup, and borscht.

- Pickles, smoked meats, marinades, spicy and salty dishes, and spicy seasonings.

- Canned meat, fish and other snack foods, plus smoked sausage.

- Cold and carbonated drinks.

- Chocolate, cocoa, and ice cream.

- Alcohol in all forms.

- White cabbage, legumes, spinach, sorrel, mushrooms, radishes, rutabaga, onions, garlic, spices; foods rich in organic acids: acidic varieties of berries and fruits - cranberries, gooseberries, red and black currants, red cherries, lemons, and acidic varieties of apples.

5.1.1.4 Approximate One-Day Diet Menu

- 1st breakfast: steam protein omelet, buckwheat porridge mashed without sugar, and tea with milk.

- 2nd breakfast: meatballs, baked apple without sugar.

- Lunch: mashed pearl barley soup with carrots, steamed meat patties with carrot puree, and dried fruit compote mashed (on xylitol).

- Snack: cottage cheese pudding without sugar.

- Dinner: boiled fish with mashed potatoes, meatloaf, and tea.

- For the whole day: white bread - 300g, sugar - 40g.

- At lunch, the third dish is served unsweetened (without sugar) or on xylitol (10-15g per serving), using other sugar substitutes.

- Sugar in the hands of the patient is given in limited quantities

5.2 After Surgery on the Stomach and Duodenum

In the first after surgical treatment, nutrition is carried out according to the principles of parenteral and enteral artificial nutrition.

In the future, when transferring the patient to outpatient treatment, a wiped version of the diet N°5f is prescribed, which helps to reduce inflammation in the gastrointestinal tract and improve postoperative healing processes. This diet is the basis for preventing the development of complications and the adverse course of the disease. Such nutrition is carried out 2–4 months after surgery.

Then, after 2–4 months (in some patients after 4–5 months), it is recommended to switch to an unapproved diet of diet N°5f, which helps to further adapt the functioning of the gastrointestinal tract and the whole body after a surgical injury. It has a beneficial effect on the activity of the liver, biliary tract, pancreas, and intestines. The transition from mashed to non-mashed diet should be done gradually.

In the first days, non-mashed vegetables are recommended in a small quantity. First, they give non-mashed vegetables in the first dish, and later add black bread, sauerkraut, and salads. Changing the diet can only be carried out with good dynamics of rehabilitation treatment. It is advisable to follow an unprotected diet N°5f for a sufficiently long time (in some cases for many years) since the restoration of the functional state of the digestive organs occurs gradually and sometimes very slowly.

However, after 1–1.5 years after surgery, in the absence of complications from the digestive system, the patient's nutrition expands to a more balanced diet. It is important to observe the principle of fractional nutrition, and it is necessary to limit the consumption of foods and dishes that are poorly intolerant to patients.

Patients who have undergone surgery on their stomachs are advised to follow a fractional diet (4–5 times a day), limit foods and dishes that most often cause dumping syndrome (sugary drinks, sweet milk porridge, very hot and very cold dishes throughout their lives), and take food slowly, chewing it carefully.

5.3   Post-Gastroresection Syndromes

Among the adverse effects of operations on the stomach, the following pathological conditions are distinguished:

- Dumping syndrome
- Afferent loop syndrome
- Asthenic syndrome
- Enteral Syndrome
- Peptic ulcer anastomosis
- Gastritis of the stomach stump

5.3.1 Dumping Syndrome

Dumping syndrome is the most common complication that occurs at various times after gastrectomy for peptic ulcer disease.

The main signs of this disease are fever, palpitations, shortness of breath, sweating, weakness, dizziness, dry mouth, nausea, vomiting, "lightheadedness," abdominal pain, bloating, diarrhea, drowsiness, fatigue, irresistible desire to lie down, and fainting. All these phenomena appear most often after eating, especially after eating sweet, hot, dairy food. When lying down, these phenomena are weakened.

The occurrence of dumping syndrome is associated with a rapid transition (discharge) of insufficiently digested food from the stomach stump directly into the small intestine, bypassing the duodenum removed during the operation.

The rapid passage of chyme through the small intestine provokes violations of humoral regulation due to changes in the intracretory function of the pancreas. As a result, pathological manifestations of dumping syndrome occur.

5.3.1.1 Degrees of Dumping Syndrome

There are three degrees of severity of dumping syndrome;

- Mild severity: it is characterized by the fact that seizures occur only after an abundant intake of food or food rich in simple carbohydrates. The attack is accompanied by mild vasomotor and intestinal symptoms, which quickly pass in the patient's lying position. Disability in these patients persists.

- The moderate severity of dumping syndrome: it manifests itself as severe vasomotor disorders and intestinal symptoms that occur daily. The patient is forced to take a horizontal position, which improves his health. The overall performance of the patient is reduced.

- A severe form of dumping syndrome: it manifests itself in pronounced seizures after almost every meal, sometimes with a swoon, which puts the patient in bed for 1–2 hours. The disability of patients is sharply reduced or completely lost. The leading treatment for dumping syndrome is an adequately constructed diet program.

5.3.1.2 General Nutrition Guidelines

Frequent fractional meals in small portions (5-7 times a day). Eat slowly. Food should be chewed slowly and thoroughly.

- Restriction of foods and dishes that most often cause dumping syndrome: sweets (sugar, honey, jam), very hot or very cold dishes, liquid sweet milk porridges, etc.

- Fluids should be taken separately from other dishes, i.e., tea, milk, the third dish at lunch and kefir in the evening should be consumed 20-30 minutes after the main meal. The amount of fluid at one time should not be plentiful (no more than 1 glass).

- Food and drinks should be warm.

- After eating, the patient should take a lying position for 20-30 minutes, especially after lunch.

- Food should contain a sufficient amount of pectin (vegetables and fruits).

5.3.1.3 Stages of Diet Therapy

In the first after surgical treatment, nutrition is carried out according to the principles of parenteral and enteral artificial nutrition.

In the future, when transferring the patient to outpatient treatment, a wiped version of the diet N°5f is prescribed, which helps to reduce inflammation in the gastrointestinal tract and improve postoperative healing processes. This diet is the basis for preventing the development of complications and the adverse course of the disease. Such nutrition is carried out 4-6 months after surgery.

Then, after 4-6 (or more) months, it is recommended to switch to diet N°5. At the same time, foods and dishes containing simple (quickly absorbed) carbohydrates — sweet liquid milk cereals, especially semolina, rice, sweet milk, and sweet tea — are sharply limited in nutrition. Cold and very hot dishes are contraindicated for patients. Separate intake of a liquid and a dense part of the diet is recommended; moreover, the liquid should be consumed 30 minutes after the ingestion of solid food, and during lunch, the second dish must be eaten first, and then the first one can be eaten.

With positive dynamics, after 1.5-2 years, the patient is transferred to a more balanced and varied diet, taking in account the principles of fragmentation of nutrition and restriction of foods and dishes that provoke dumping syndrome.

For complications of pancreatitis dumping syndrome or suspected peptic ulcer of a stomach stump, anastomosis, or jejunum, diet N°1 is recommended with the addition of a protein dish at 5 p.m. In the absence of complications and with good health of the patient, the diet can be gradually expanded, observing its basic principles, and gradually switch to a normal diet.

5.3.2 Afferent Loop Syndrome

The pathogenesis of the lead loop syndrome is based on a violation of the evacuation of contents from the lead loop due to its excesses, adhesions, and impaired motor function due to changes in normal anatomical relationships.

Loopback syndrome usually develops during the first year after surgery. It is manifested by severe pain in the epigastrium and right hypochondrium, and vomiting of bile after eating. In between meals, patients experience a feeling of heaviness in the upper abdomen as a result of throwing intestinal contents back into the stomach, the accumulation of fluid and food in the afferent loop and the cult of the stomach.

The strategies of restorative treatment and clinical nutrition for the adherent loop syndrome are the same as for dumping syndrome.

5.3.3 Asthenic Syndrome

Asthenic syndrome is a late postoperative complication of gastric resection.

The frequency of its appearance is in direct proportion to the level of resection of the stomach. Of great importance in the pathogenesis of this condition is a violation of the secretory and motor functions of the stump of the resected stomach, a change in the secretion of bile and pancreatic juice. In pathogenesis, rapid passage through the jejunum, impaired absorption of iron and vitamins, are of particular importance.

Patients are characterized by rapid fatigue, general malaise, weight loss, signs of hypovitaminosis, a tendency to hypotension and fainting conditions, and neuropsychic disorders. General weakness intensifies most often after eating, especially rich in carbohydrates. There are various dyspeptic phenomena: decreased appetite, belching, regurgitation with a bitter fluid, and a feeling of heaviness in the epigastric region.

A characteristic symptom is a disorder of intestinal activity, expressed in the appearance (especially after milk and fatty foods) of loud intestinal sounds and diarrhea.

Dietary recommendations for a patient with agastral asthenia consist of the appointment of a high-protein diet N°1c. Products that are not tolerated by patients are excluded from the diet, and the diet is also enriched with specialized protein-vitamin products, mixtures for enteral nutrition, and high-calorie diet products.

5.3.4 Peptic Ulcers of the Anastomosis and Gastritis of the Gastric Stump

In the mechanisms of development of peptic ulcers of the anastomosis and gastritis of the gastric stump, paramount importance is given to the aggressive effect of gastric juice and the development of Helicobacter pylori infection. In addition, it is important that the duodenal and intestinal contents are thrown into the stomach, the weak peristaltic function of the stomach stump, and its rapid emptying after eating.

The clinic of peptic ulcer of the anastomosis is similar to the manifestations of peptic ulcer, but the symptoms of the disease are usually more intense, the periods of exacerbation are longer than with the ulcer, for which the operation was performed. It is characterized by a decrease in appetite and weight loss.

Patients should be transferred to the wiped version of diet N°1c, with an increased amount of protein. The mashed diet is prescribed before the exacerbation subsides (sometimes for a sufficiently long period of up to 2-3 months). In the future, patients can be recommended non-rubbed version of diet N°1c.

5.4 After Bowel Surgery

Proper diet therapy after intestinal surgery helps to reduce the incidence of complications and more quickly recover the patient.

Traditional approaches of clinical nutrition for patients who underwent surgery on the small and large intestines, based only on the principles of balanced nutrition, do not lead to the restoration of the entire volume of physiological functions. It is advisable to approach the rehabilitation of patients after intestinal resection, from the standpoint of the theory of adequate nutrition. It is necessary to ensure that not only the elemental restoration of nutrients in the body but also to maximize the restoration of cavity and membrane digestion, absorption in the intestine, as well as restore normal micro biogenesis. Only under these conditions that normalization of the entire digestive tract is possible.

5.4.1 Principles

- Clinical nutrition should provide sparing of the intestine, as well as other parts of the gastrointestinal tract.

- Clinical nutrition should help normalize metabolism and restore the body.

- Clinical nutrition should increase the body's resistance to inflammation and intoxication.

- Clinical nutrition should contribute to the healing of the surgical wound.

- In the absence of complications, an earlier transfer of patients to physiologically complete nutrition with a wide grocery set is desirable.

5.4.2 Stage of Diet Therapy after Bowel Surgery

In the immediate postoperative period, it is necessary to establish the parenteral nutrition of the patient. First of all, this concerns the introduction of energy substrates. The volume and composition of parenteral nutrition are determined individually, depending on the needs of the patient.

Stabilization of the patient and controlled diarrhea are indications of the transition to nutrition using the gastrointestinal tract. This usually occurs 3-4 days after surgery. At the same time, with extensive resections of the small intestine, some experts recommend starting enteral nutrition 2–4 weeks after surgery. In most clinical cases, standard enteral nutrition mixtures are prescribed; however, for resection of the small intestine, it is advisable to use semi-liquid food products. Combined parenteral-enteral nutrition in the comprehensive rehabilitation of patients after surgical interventions in the intestine can reduce the time and increase the effectiveness of rehabilitation treatment, significantly reduce the frequency of complications and adverse outcomes of the postoperative process.

With the positive dynamics of the patient's condition, a transition to natural nutrition is recommended. However, it should be remembered that the unreasonably early transfer of patients to natural nutrition after operations on the intestine significantly worsens the course of the recovery period, stimulates the development of enteric insufficiency syndrome, and disrupts the natural mechanisms of cavity and membrane digestion.

After artificial nutrition, patients are assigned a low caloric diet. This diet is characterized by an extremely low nutritional value (750-800 kcal), and the patient's body experiences nutritional hunger during the entire time of its use. As a result of this, tissue repair mechanisms are significantly inhibited, and conditions are created for the formation of an unfavorable course of the disease. Therefore, dietary treatment using low caloric diet requires simultaneous parallel parenteral nutrition of patients.

With good tolerance of the low caloric diet and the absence of diarrhea, after 2-3 days, patients should be transferred to diet N°1a. It is prescribed for 2–4 days after the low caloric diet. However, if there are opportunities for parenteral nutrition (transfusion of protein-energy mixtures) and in the presence of at least minimally expressed diarrhea, the appointment of diet N°1a should be postponed for several days.

With good tolerance of diet N°1a, the patient is transferred to diet N°1b.

Typically, by 14-15 days after surgery on the intestines, it is recommended that the main diet N°1 be prescribed. At the same time, the patient should adhere to the wiped version of the diet, even after transferring to outpatient treatment.

3-4 weeks after the patient's discharge from the hospital, a gradual transition to the non-rubbed version of diet N°1 is required. The gradual change from one version of the diet to another involves a daily decrease in the number of dishes. The good tolerance of the introduced dishes is evidence of the normalization of the secretory and motor-evacuation functions of the digestive system and allows to continue the expansion of the diet.

With positive dynamics after 5-6 weeks, the patient is transferred to a more balanced and varied diet.

If patients tolerate milk poorly after intestinal surgery, milk consumption should be excluded for a long time (sometimes forever). Lactose overload in the presence of enzyme deficiency can aggravate secretory disorders of the intestine. Thus, with the development of postoperative lactose deficiency in the diet of patients, whole milk should be maximally and permanently limited. This applies to a lesser extent to the consumption of lactic acid products. The replacement of dairy products can be successfully carried out due to soy products. Soy proteins are a vital source of additional support for the body with a highly plastic protein.

5.4.3 Short Bowel Syndrome

A condition that develops after resection of the small intestine and is characterized by diarrhea, steatorrhea, and malabsorption of nutrients is commonly called short (or shortened) bowel syndrome.

When less than 50% of the small intestine is removed, the syndrome of the small intestine proceeds subclinically, but a larger volume of resection leads to increasing diarrhea, steatorrhea, iron, and folic acid deficiency.

In patients with a favorable course of the postoperative period with fairly rapid restoration of intestinal functions, a gradual, but reasonably quick transition to complete natural nutrition should be carried out. However, after extensive intestinal resections, the transition from complete parenteral to natural nutrition should go through a fairly long stage of partial parenteral nutrition, sometimes stretched for several months. The duration of the transition period is determined purely individually. In some cases, with extensive resections of the small intestine, the patient must receive full or partial parenteral nutrition for life.

The introduction of new products in the diet should strictly depend on the individual tolerance of patients. Protein-energy deficiency of the diets in relation to the physiological needs of the body should be covered by parenteral nutrition. The sequence of application of standard diets is given above.

After switching to full natural nutrition, patients with a small intestine are recommended a diet with a high content of protein, carbohydrates, and a moderate amount of fat. The diet should be supplemented with triglycerides with an average carbon chain length, multivitamins in liquid forms, vitamin B_{12} (intramuscularly 1mg every 2-4 weeks), folic acid (intramuscularly 15mg per week), vitamin K (intramuscularly 10mg per week), iron preparations (parenteral and then oral).

Dynamic laboratory monitoring of urinary oxalate levels is required. When the first signs of hyperoxaluria appear, it is necessary to limit the intake of products containing an increased amount of oxalates (sorrel, spinach, parsley, potatoes, and chocolate).

1-2 years after the operation, various clinical options for the course of the disease can be observed. Depending on the condition of the patient, a nutritional program is prescribed.

The following individual scenarios of patient diet therapy are possible:

- Natural normal or near-normal nutrition.

- Natural nutrition using individually selected specialized foods containing depolymerized (short-beaked) nutrients (proteins, fats, and carbohydrates).

- Natural nutrition with partial parenteral support.

- Complete parenteral nutrition.

5.5 After Surgery on the Liver

In the immediate postoperative period, it is necessary to establish the parenteral nutrition of the patient. First of all, this concerns the introduction of energy substrates. The volume and composition of parenteral nutrition are determined individually, depending on the needs of the patient. The currently recommended duration of a complete balanced (for proteins, fats, carbohydrates) parenteral nutrition depends on the volume and complexity of the operation on the liver and is, on average, 3-5 days.

The transition to natural nutrition should go through the stage of combined (parenteral-enteral) nutrition lasting at least 4-5 days. This is due to the fact that as a result of liver injury, there is significant inhibition of the function of the small intestine, the restoration of which takes at least 7-10 days after surgery. Probe introduction of elemental nutrient mixtures into the digestive system is gradually increasing quantities will ensure in patients after liver operations, the adaptation of the gastrointestinal tract to increasing nutritional loads. The combination of enteral nutrition with parenteral nutrition is aimed at preventing metabolic hunger.

For small amounts of surgery 7-10 days after surgery, it is advisable to recommend a diet N°5d (sparing) or diet N°5a. After 3-4 weeks, with good tolerance, the patient is recommended to switch to diet N°5. Usually, this happens already at the outpatient stage of treatment.

5.6 After Surgery on the Biliary Tract
5.6.1 General Nutritional Guidelines

- Frequent, fractional nutrition. Eating every 3.5-4 hours.

- Limit cholesterol-rich foods.

- Uniform distribution of fats for all meals and mixing them with food, which contributes to better absorption of fats, prevention of pain and dyspeptic phenomena.

After operations on the biliary tract, the tolerability of so many products deteriorates, which requires minimizing their use. Especially, ill patients tolerate vegetables rich in essential oils (radish, radish, and green onions), spicy dishes (peppers, marinades, mayonnaise, and canned food). Also, patients who underwent surgery on the biliary tract, often poorly perceive milk, ice cream, chocolate, and cocoa.

5.6.2 Cholecystectomy

1st-day hunger.

24 hours after surgery - mineral water without gas or broth of wild rose without sugar (in small sips, not more than 1 liter per day).

After 36–48 hours - mineral water without gas, unsweetened dried fruit jelly, unsweetened weak tea, low-fat kefir in a volume of 1–1.5l during the day (100–150ml per dose every three hours).

On the 2nd – 4th day, low caloric diet. On the 5-7th day, diet N°1a and diet N°1b are sequential. In diets N°1a and 1b for patients who underwent cholecystectomy, only mucous soups, eggs in the form of steam protein omelets are used.

On the 8–10th day after the operation, with an uncomplicated course of the disease and good tolerance of the ongoing diet therapy, the diet N°5a is prescribed.

In the future, the transition to an unprotected version of diet N°5a is carried out. It is recommended to follow this diet for 1.5–2 months after cholecystectomy and other types of surgical treatment of diseases of the biliary system.

However, not all patients tolerate diet N°5a well: transient diarrhea, bloating, flatulence, and the appearance of pain associated with this in the pyloroduodenal zone and right hypochondrium occur. For these cases, a diet N°5d (sparing) has been developed, this diet is also prescribed for 1–1.5 months after surgery on the biliary tract. However, diet N°5d (sparing) is not indicated for patients with reduced body weight due to its low energy intensity. Moreover, the complete exclusion of vegetable oil against the background of a sharp restriction of fats can contribute to the development of the cholestatic syndrome.

Failure to comply with the principle of biochemical and mechanical sparing of the digestive system in 1.5–2 months of rehabilitation treatment after cholecystectomy can lead to the formation of a chronic course of enteric insufficiency as a form of postcholecystectomy syndrome.

In the future, when restoring the physiological functions of the body, diet N°5 is prescribed. Compliance with diet N°5 with good tolerability is recommended for patients for 1.5–2 years. Diet N°5 should be individualized. Particular attention should be paid to the tolerance of products containing animal fats, some vegetables, sweet dishes, eggs, and dishes from them, milk, and some juices. When there are disorders associated with the intake of certain products, in violation of the planed diet, patients need to review the diet. In the future, patients are assigned a diet N°1.

5.6.3 Postcholecystectomy Syndrome

In 20–40% of patients after cholecystectomy, a postcholecystectomy syndrome develops. A wide variety of diseases can cause this syndrome: stones in the bile ducts, spasm or stricture of the sphincter of Oddi, gastritis, duodenitis, peptic ulcer, pancreatitis, and intestinal dysbiosis. It is necessary to clarify the cause of postcholecystectomy syndrome, and then prescribe medication and dietary treatment.

With postcholecystectomy syndrome, the following diets are used:

- With an exacerbation of the disease - diet N°5d, diet N°5.

- In a state of remission - diet N°5.

- If bile stasis, hypomotor dyskinesia occurs after cholecystectomy, use the diet N°5e (lipotropic fat).

5.7 After Pancreatic Surgery

The clinical nutrition for patients undergoing pancreatic surgery, regardless of the nature of the disease, should consist of two stages: artificial nutrition (parenteral, probe, mixed) and natural nutrition.

The outcome of surgery is positively affected by the duration of the patient's artificial nutrition, adequate component composition, and energy value of nutritional support.

5.7.1 Phase of Diet Therapy

- The first stage is to complete parenteral nutrition. The duration of complete parenteral nutrition of patients who underwent severe surgical interventions on the pancreas should be at least 10–12 days, provided that the protein and energy supply of nutritional support is complete. This allows to minimize postoperative complications. With less severe surgical interventions, the transition from parenteral to natural nutrition can take place no earlier than the 5-7th day.

- The second stage is partial parenteral nutrition. It is used during the transition to natural nutrition. The combination of a gradually increasing volume of natural nutrition with gradually reducing parenteral nutrition is the main requirement for clinical nutrition in the conditions of postoperative rehabilitation. This allows to maintain at the proper physiological level the protein-energy supply of the body during this period of rehabilitation and, at the same time, carry out a smoothly increasing nutritional load due to the mechanically, biochemically, and thermally sparing hypocaloric diet.

- The third stage is natural nutrition. It is necessary to increase the nutritional load of patients as slowly as possible after operations on the pancreas. Addressing the expansion of the diet, the transition from one diet to another requires a thorough assessment of indicators of the state of the body and the characteristics of the disease.

- Initially, after pancreatic surgery, patients are prescribed a low caloric diet for a period of 5–7 days, and not for 2–3 days, as with operations on other organs.

- To replace the low caloric diet, diet N°1a is prescribed for a period of 5–7 days, also compensating for the protein-energy deficiency through parenteral nutrition.

- In the future, it is recommended to switch to diet N°1b for 5-7 days.

- In the future, the first version of diet N°5c is prescribed. It is used for 1.5–2 months.

Then, for 6-12 months, the second version of diet N°5c is used. With good health, this diet is expanded with the gradual inclusion of new products, dishes, and an increase in their volume. In the absence of diarrhea, the diet includes raw, finely chopped vegetables (carrots, cabbage), taken 3-4 times a day at the beginning of a meal, 100-150g. With the development of secretory and endocrine pancreatic insufficiency in the postoperative period, there are symptoms of pancreatogenic enteropathy (diarrhea, steatorrhea, and malabsorption) with the development of protein-energy deficiency. This category of patients requires an increase in protein intake to 120–130g and a decrease to 60–70g of fat. Non-fat meat (veal, rabbit meat, chickens), low-fat dairy products, fish, egg white are used as a source of protein. Eliminate fiber-rich foods. Products are introduced into the diet, rich in salts of potassium (carrot and other juices before meals, stewed fruit pureed), and calcium (calcined and unleavened cottage cheese). The diet is supplemented with multivitamin preparations or vitamin-mineral complexes. It is advisable to include in the diet modular protein enteral mixtures, homogenized and purees canned foods for children and diet food. In the case of impaired glucose tolerance or the development of diabetes, they exclude from the diet or significantly limit the intake of easily digestible carbohydrates, homogenized and mashed canned foods for children, and diet food.

TECHNICAL DIET MODELS FOR DIGESTIVE DISEASES

6.1 Diet N°1

Peptic ulcer of the stomach and duodenum in the stage of decaying exacerbation, during recovery and remission (duration of dietary treatment 3-5 months), acute gastritis during recovery and in the phase of convalescence, chronic gastritis with secretory insufficiency in the acute phase, chronic gastritis with normal and increased secretion (the duration of dietary treatment is 3-5 months until the exacerbation is completely stopped).

Esophagus diseases: esophagitis, gastroesophageal reflux disease (GERD).

6.1.1 Objectives

Acceleration of repair processes of ulcers and erosion, further reduction or prevention of inflammation of the gastric mucosa and duodenum.

This diet helps to normalize the secretory and motor-evacuation functions of the stomach.

Diet N°1 is designed to meet the physiological needs of the body for nutrients in stationary conditions or on an outpatient basis during work that is not associated with physical activity.

6.1.2 General characteristics

The use of diet N°1 is aimed at providing moderate gastric sparing from mechanical, chemical, and temperature aggression with a restriction in the diet of dishes that have a pronounced irritant effect on the walls and receptor apparatus of the upper gastrointestinal tract, as well as indigestible products. Exclude dishes that are strong causative agents of secretion and chemically irritating the gastric mucosa. Both very hot and very cold dishes are excluded from the diet.

The rationing of diet N°1 is fractional, up to 6 times a day, in small portions. The interval between meals mustn't be more than 4 hours, one hour before bedtime light dinner is allowed. At night a glass of milk or cream can be drunk. It is recommended to chew food carefully.

The food is liquid, mushy and of a more dense consistency in a boiled and mostly mashed form. Since the consistency of the food is vital in clinical nutrition, they reduce the amount of fiber-rich foods (such as turnip, radish, radish, asparagus, beans, and peas), peeled fruits and unripe berries with a rough skin (such as gooseberries, currants, grapes, dates), bread made from wholemeal flour, and products containing coarse connective tissue (such as cartilage, skin of poultry and fish, sinewy meat).

Dishes are cooked, boiled or steamed. After that, they are crushed to a mushy state. Fish and lean meats can be consumed as a whole. Some dishes can be baked but without a crust.

6.1.3 Composition

Proteins 100g (of which 60% is of animal origin), fats 90-100g (30% vegetable), carbohydrates 400g, sodium chloride 6g, calorie content 2800-2900kcal, ascorbic acid 100mg, retinol 2mg, thiamine 4mg, Riboflavin 4mg; Nicotinic acid 30mg; calcium 0.8g, phosphorus not less than 1.6g, magnesium 0.5g, iron 15mg. The total amount of free liquid is 1.5 liters; the food temperature is normal. Salt is recommended to limit.

6.1.4 Recommended foods

- Wheat bread from yesterday's highest grade flour or dried; rye bread and any fresh bread, pastry and puff pastry are excluded.

- Soups on a vegetable broth from mashed and well-boiled cereals, dairy, mashed soups from vegetables, seasoned with butter, egg and milk mixture, cream; meat and fish broths, mushroom and strong vegetable broths, cabbage soup, borscht, and okroshka are excluded.

- Meat dishes - steamed and boiled from beef, young low-fat mutton, edged pork, chicken, turkey; fatty and sinewy varieties of meat, poultry, duck, goose, canned meat, smoked foods are excluded.

- Dishes from fish are usually low-fat varieties, without skin, in a piece or the form of cutlets; cooked in water or steam.

- Dairy products - milk, cream, non-acidic kefir, yogurt, cottage cheese in the form of soufflé, lazy dumplings, and pudding. High acidity dairy products are excluded.

- Porridge made from semolina, buckwheat, rice, boiled in water, milk, semi-viscous, mashed; millet, pearl barley, and barley groats, legumes, pasta are excluded.

- Vegetables - potatoes, carrots, beets, cauliflower, cooked in water or steam, in the form of soufflé, mashed potatoes, and steam puddings.

- Snacks - a salad of boiled vegetables, a tongue from a barbecue, a doctor's sausage, dairy, dietary, and jellied fish on a vegetable broth.

- Sweet dishes - fruit puree, jelly, mashed compotes, sugar, and honey.

- Drinks - weak tea with milk, cream, sweet juices from fruits and berries.

- Fats - butter and refined sunflower oil, added to dishes.

6.1.5 Excluded foods

Two groups of foods should be excluded from this diet.

- Products that cause or intensify the pain. These include: drinks - strong tea, coffee, carbonated drinks; tomatoes, and others.

- Products that strongly stimulate the secretion of the stomach and intestines. These include concentrated meat and fish broths, decoctions of mushrooms; fried foods; meat and fish stewed in their own juice; meat, fish, tomato and mushroom sauces; salted or smoked fish and meat products; canned meat and fish; salted, pickled vegetables and fruits; spices and seasonings (mustard, horseradish).

In addition, the following are excluded: rye and any fresh bread, pastry; high acidity dairy products; millet, pearl barley, and corn grits, legumes; white cabbage, radish, sorrel, onions, cucumbers; salted, pickled and pickled vegetables, mushrooms; sour and fiber-rich fruits and berries.

It is necessary to focus on the patient's sensations. If, when eating a certain product, the patient feels discomfort in the epigastric region, and especially nausea, vomiting, then this product should be discarded.

6.1.6 Diet Sample for a week

Monday

- First breakfast: soft-boiled egg, milk porridge, tea with milk.
- Second breakfast: fresh non-acidic cottage cheese, rosehip broth.
- Lunch: milk oat soup, steamed meatballs with carrot puree, fruit mousse.
- Snack: broth of wild rose, crackers.
- Dinner: boiled fish, baked with milk sauce, mashed potatoes, tea with milk.
- At night: milk.

Tuesday

- First breakfast: steam omelet, loose buckwheat porridge, tea with milk.
- Second breakfast: baked apple with sugar.
- Lunch: milk rice soup, steam souffle with mashed potatoes, apple jelly.
- Snack: a decoction of wheat bran with sugar and crackers.
- Dinner: steamed soufflé and fruit jelly.
- At night: cream.

Wednesday

- First breakfast: soft-boiled egg, milk semolina, and kissel.
- Lunch: curd pudding.
- Lunch: vegetarian potato soup, boiled meat, baked with bechamel sauce, boiled carrots, and stewed boiled, dried fruit compote.
- Snack: broth of wild rose, inedible bun.
- Dinner: boiled fish, baked with milk sauce, carrot and apple roll, and tea with milk.
- At night: milk.

Thursday

- First breakfast: lazy dumplings with non-sour cream, oatmeal porridge, and stewed fruit.
- Second breakfast: fresh non-acidic cottage cheese and rosehip broth.
- Lunch: milk soup with noodles, dumplings from turkey meat with a side dish of boiled cauliflower, weak tea with milk.
- Snack: a decoction of wheat bran with a dry biscuit.
- Dinner: a salad of boiled vegetables and boiled sausages, berry mousse, and jelly.
- At night: cream.

Friday

- First breakfast: soft-boiled egg and milk porridge.
- Lunch: baked pear with sugar and dried fruit compote.
- Lunch: mashed soup from vegetables, boiled pike perch, vermicelli, and weak tea.
- Snack: berry mousse.
- Dinner: meat souffle, cottage cheese casserole, and jelly.
- At night: milk.

Saturday

- First breakfast: steam omelet, semolina porridge, and dried fruit compote.
- Second breakfast: fresh, non-acidic cottage cheese and rosehip broth.
- Lunch: oat milk soup, boiled rabbit, mashed potatoes, and weak tea with milk.
- Snack: a decoction of wheat bran with a dry biscuit.
- Dinner: boiled fish baked with milk sauce, carrot and apple roll, and jelly.
- At night: cream.

Sunday

- First breakfast: steam omelet, vermicelli with grated cheese, weak tea, and meringue.

- Second breakfast: berry jelly and compote.

- Lunch: mashed vegetable soup, boiled carp with bechamel sauce, boiled rice, and jelly.

- Snack: cottage cheese casserole and weak tea.

- Dinner: vegetable salad and meatballs from turkey meat with a side dish of cauliflower.

- At night: milk.

6.1.7 Variants and Options

For the treatment of patients with peptic ulcer in adolescence, they recommend the option of diet N°1, in which the protein content is increased by 20g and fat by 30g. Accordingly, the calorie content increases to 3160kcal.

With gastritis, the diet is determined by the stage of the disease, the severity of the clinical manifestations. So, with acute gastritis on the 1st day, the patient should refrain from eating; on the 2nd day, mucous soup, jelly, meat souffle, rosehip broth are prescribed; on the 3rd day - white crackers, steam cutlets, meatballs, weak broth, and mashed vegetables. With the extinction of acute phenomena of the disease, the patient is transferred to diet N°1.

In chronic gastritis with increased or preserved secretion, the diet is the same as with peptic ulcers.

In chronic gastritis with secretory insufficiency, frequent, fractional nutrition is necessary, subject to mechanical sparing of the gastric mucosa and chemical stimulation by food irritants of its glandular apparatus (diet N°2).

6.1.7.1 Diet N°1a

This diet is recommended to maximize the restriction of mechanical, chemical, and temperature aggression on the stomach. This diet is prescribed for exacerbation of peptic ulcer, bleeding, acute gastritis, and other diseases that require maximum gastric sparing. Diet N°1a is also prescribed for exacerbation of peptic ulcer in patients undergoing cholecystectomy. Diet N°1a is prescribed in the first days of treatment (but not longer than 7-14 days). After that, they switch to diet N°1b (more stressful).

6.1.7.1.1 Purpose

Reducing the reflex excitability of the stomach, reducing the interoceptive irritations emanating from the affected organ, and restoring the mucous membrane by maximizing the gastric function.

6.1.7.1.2 General characteristics

Exclusion of substances that are strong causative agents of secretion, as well as mechanical, chemical, and thermal stimuli. Food is prepared only in liquid and mushy form. Steam, boiled, and mashed dishes in a liquid or gruel-like consistency. In diet N°1a for patients undergoing cholecystectomy, only mucous soups, eggs in the form of steam protein omelets are used. Calorie is reduced mainly due to carbohydrates. The amount of food taken at one time is limited; the frequency of intake is at least 6 times.

6.1.7.1.3 Composition

Diet N°1a is characterized by a decrease in the content of proteins and fats to the lower limit of the physiological norm, a strict limitation of the effect of various chemical and mechanical stimuli on the upper sections of the gastrointestinal tract. With this diet, carbohydrates and salt are also limited.

Proteins 80g, fats 80-90g, carbohydrates 200g, sodium chloride 16g, calories 1800-1900kcal; retinol 2mg, thiamine 4mg, riboflavin 4mg, nicotinic acid 30mg, ascorbic acid 100mg; calcium 0.8g, phosphorus 1.6g, magnesium 0.5g, and iron 0.015g. The temperature of hot dishes is not higher than 50-55 °C, cold ones - not lower than 15-20 °C.

6.1.7.1.4 Recommended foods

- Mucous soups from semolina, oat, rice, pearl barley with the addition of egg-milk mixture, cream, and butter.

- Meat and poultry dishes in the form of mashed potatoes or steam soufflé (meat cleared of tendons, fascia, and skin is passed 2-3 times through a meat grinder).

- Fish dishes in the form of a steam soufflé from low-fat varieties.

- Dairy products - milk, cream, steam souffle from freshly prepared mashed cottage cheese; sour-milk drinks, cheese, sour cream, and ordinary cottage cheese are excluded. With good tolerance, they drink whole milk up to 2–4 times a day.

- Soft-boiled eggs or in the form of a steam omelet, no more than 2 per day.

- Dishes from cereals in the form of liquid cereal in milk, cereal from cereal (buckwheat, oatmeal) flour with the addition of milk or cream. Almost all cereals can be used, except for pearl barley and millet. Butter is added to the finished porridge.

- Sweet dishes - jelly and jelly from sweet berries and fruits, sugar, honey. Juices from berries and fruits can be prepared, diluting them before taking boiled water at a ratio of 1:1.

- Fats - fresh butter and vegetable oil added to dishes.

- Drinks: weak tea with milk or cream, juices from fresh berries, fruits, diluted with water. Of the drinks, broths of wild rose and wheat bran are especially useful.

6.1.7.1.5 Excluded foods

Bread and bakery products; broths; fried foods; mushrooms; smoked meats; fatty and spicy dishes; vegetable dishes; various snacks; coffee, cocoa, strong tea; vegetable juices, concentrated fruit juices; sour-milk and carbonated drinks; sauces (ketchup, vinegar, mayonnaise) and spices.

Approximate one-day diet menu (option for patients after cholecystectomy)

- 1st breakfast: liquid mashed oatmeal on the water - 200g with milk and 5g butter, a steam protein omelet from 2 eggs, and tea with lemon.

- 2nd breakfast: fat-free cottage cheese, rosehip broth - 100g.

- Lunch: mucous soup with semolina - 200g, steamed souffle from boiled meat - 50g, broth of compote - 100g.

- Snack: mashed meat - 50g, milk cream - 150g, rosehip broth - 100g.

- Dinner: steamed fish soufflé, liquid mashed buckwheat katana in water - 200g with milk and 5g butter, tea with lemon.

- At night: fruit jelly - 150g, rosehip broth - 100g.

- For the whole day: butter - 20g, sugar - 40g.

6.1.7.2 Diet N°1b

Indications and intended use for diet N°1a in fractional meals (6 times a day) is for less severe, in comparison with table N°1a, restrictions on mechanical, chemical, and temperature aggression on the stomach. This diet is indicated for a mild exacerbation of peptic ulcer of the stomach or duodenum, at the stage of calming down this process, with chronic gastritis.

Diet N°1b is prescribed in the subsequent stages of treatment with the patient remaining in bed. Duration of diet N°1b is very individual, but on average, they range from 10 to 30 days. Diet N°1b is also used subject to bed rest. The difference from diet N°1a is a gradual increase in the content of basic nutrients and caloric intake.

Bread is allowed in the form of dried (but unroasted) crackers (75-100g). Rubbed mucous soups are introduced; milk porridge can be consumed more often. Homogenized canned foods for baby foods made from fruits and vegetables and beaten egg dishes are allowed. All the recommended products and dishes of meat and fish are given in the form of steam soufflé, knives, mashed potatoes, and cutlets. After the products are boiled to softness, they are rubbed into a mushy state. The food should be warm. The remaining recommendations are the same as for diet N°1a.

6.1.7.2.1 Composition

Proteins up to 100g, fats up to 100g (30g vegetable), carbohydrates 300g, calorie content 2300-2500kcal, table salt 6g; retinol 2mg, thiamine 4mg, riboflavin 4mg, nicotinic acid 30mg, ascorbic acid

100mg; calcium 0.8g, phosphorus 1.2g, magnesium 0.5g, iron 15mg. The total amount of free fluid is 2 liters. The temperature of hot dishes is up to 55-60 °C, of cold ones - not lower than 15-20 °C.

6.1.7.3 Diet N°1c

The main indication for its appointment is peptic ulcer disease with an unfavorable, severe course, metabolic disorders.

6.1.7.3.1 Purpose

Gastric sparing by limiting mechanical, chemical, and thermal stimuli, stimulating healing processes in the mucous membrane, increasing its protective capabilities, and enhancing the anti-inflammatory effect of treatment.

6.1.7.3.2 General characteristics

A physiologically complete diet with high protein content increased (compared with diet N°1) the content of fats and fiber, vitamins. It provides stimulation of protein metabolism, normalization of the motor-evacuation function of the gastrointestinal tract, and the processes of its nervous regulation. Cooked and steamed dishes. Raw vegetable salads are included. The temperature of the dishes is normal. Diet should be fractionated 6-7 times a day.

6.1.7.3.3 Composition

Proteins up to 130-150g (1/3 vegetable), fats up to 130g (1/2 vegetable), carbohydrates 400g-450, calories 3600-3700kcal, sodium chloride 6g; increased amount of retinol, thiamine, riboflavin, nicotinic acid, ascorbic acid; calcium, phosphorus, magnesium, and iron. The total amount of free fluid is 1.5 liters.

6.1.7.3.4 Recommended foods

- Bread and flour products - protein bread, dry biscuits, 2-3 times a week, inedible buns and pies.

- Soups - mashed milk cereals, milk with the addition of mashed vegetables (excl. cabbage), with vermicelli and noodles; mashed vegetables.

- Meat and fish dishes - lean meats, stripped of tendons and fat in boiled and steam form, mostly chopped and in pieces. Low-fat varieties of fish in boiled and baked form; jellied meat and fish.

- Eggs - protein (from 2 eggs per day) in the form of additives, protein omelet steam.

- Dairy products - whole milk, cream; freshly prepared curd in dishes (souffle) and mashed; dairy products (kefir, one-day curdled milk, etc.).

- Vegetables and greens - various types in boiled, stewed, fresh; puddings, salads, stews, mashed potatoes, casseroles.

- Fruits and sweet foods - ripe fruits and berries (except sour varieties), in natural, baked, boiled, or mashed form. Sweet berry juices in half with water. Jam, honey, pastille, marshmallows, and marmalade.

- Cereals and pasta - mashed milk porridge (especially oatmeal, buckwheat, oatmeal), mashed steam puddings; homemade noodles, vermicelli, and finely chopped pasta.

- Fats - unsalted butter, vegetable oil (do not fry, add to dishes).

- Snacks - vinaigrettes with vegetable oil, salads from fresh vegetables and fruits, aspic, doctor's sausage, mild cheese, low-fat ham, and caviar in a small amount.

- Sauces and spices - milk, fruit sauces, sauces on a vegetable broth with leaves of parsley, dill, and sour cream.

- Drinks - weak tea with milk, cream; a decoction of wild rose and wheat bran, fruit and berry juices, and vegetable juices in half with water.

6.1.7.3.5 Excluded foods

Spicy, salty, fatty, fried foods; smoked products; canned snacks; vegetables rich in essential oils and with coarse fiber (white and red cabbage, turnips, rutabaga, radish, radishes, onions, garlic, sorrel, spinach); mushrooms and decoctions of them; alcohol; legumes (peas, beans, lentils); millet; refractory fats; raw eggs; black bread.

6.2 Diet N°2

6.2.1 Indications

Chronic gastritis with secretory insufficiency, acute gastritis during recovery, chronic enteritis and colitis after an exacerbation.

6.2.2 Purpose

Restoring the motor and secretory functions of the stomach and intestines, increasing gastric secretion, and reducing fermentation processes in the intestine. The effect of this table on the body is to exclude mechanical irritation of the stomach while maintaining chemical irritation to excite the secretory function of the stomach.

6.2.3 General characteristics

Diet N°2 is physiologically complete with the restriction of coarse fiber, free milk, spicy dishes, snacks, and spices.

Food is prepared in crushed form; during frying, the formation of a rough crust is not allowed (fried without breading).

6.2.4 Composition

Proteins 100g, fats 90g (25g vegetable), carbohydrates 400g, sodium chloride 6-8g; calorie content 2800-3000kcal; retinol 2mg, thiamine 4mg, riboflavin 4mg, nicotinic acid 30mg, ascorbic acid 100mg; calcium 0.8g, magnesium 0.5g, phosphorus 1.2g, iron 0.015g. The total amount of liquid is 1.5l. The food temperature is normal.

6.2.5 Recommended foods

It is allowed to use a wide range of dishes and products in the diet:

- Yesterday's wheat bread baking; inedible bakery products and cookies.

- Soups on weak meat, fish broth, vegetable broth with finely chopped and well-boiled vegetables or mashed cereals, noodles, with tolerance - borscht, cabbage soup from fresh cabbage.

- Non-greasy meat and poultry without fascia, tendons, or skin. It could be boiled, baked, or fried without a rough crust, as well as cutlet mass products; boiled tongue and dairy sausages.

- Fish of low-fat varieties with a piece or chopped; boiled or baked.

- Dairy products - kefir, yogurt, fresh cottage cheese in its natural form and in dishes, milk and cream, added to dishes and drinks; cheese, sour cream.

- Various cereals, except millet and pearl barley.

- Potatoes, carrots, beets, zucchini, cabbage.

- Snacks, salads from fresh tomatoes, boiled vegetables with meat, fish, or eggs.

- Soft ripe fruits and berries, in pureed form, baked apples, tangerines, oranges; watermelon, grapes without skin.

- Iris, marmalade, pastille, marshmallows, sugar, honey, jams, and preserves.

6.2.6 Excluded foods

- Fresh bread and flour products from butter and puff pastry.

- Dairy, pea, and bean soups.

- Fatty meat, poultry (duck, goose), smoked meats, canned meat and fish, fatty, salted and smoked fish.

- Raw uncooked and pickled vegetables, pickles, onions, radishes, radishes, sweet peppers, cucumbers, garlic, and mushrooms.

- Rough varieties of fruits and berries in raw form.

- Chocolate and cream products.

6.2.7 Sample diet menu for the day

- Breakfast: steam omelet, cheese, milk porridge, coffee with milk.

- Lunch: mushroom broth with cereals, boiled pike-perch with mashed potatoes, jelly.

- Snack: a decoction of wheat bran.

- Dinner: meat cutlets, fried without breading, rice pudding with fruit sauce, cocoa.

- At night: yogurt.

6.2.8 Variants and options

6.2.8.1 Diet N°2a

This diet is prescribed during the recovery period after acute colitis, enteritis, enterocolitis, gastritis, as well as chronic gastritis with secretory insufficiency and with preserved secretion.

Diet N°2a is prescribed in the absence of concomitant diseases of the liver, biliary tract, and pancreas.

Diet N°2a aims to slightly limit the mechanical and chemical stimuli that are irritating to the mucous membrane of the gastrointestinal tract. Diet N°2a is an almost complete diet containing 100g of protein, 100g of fat, and 400g of carbohydrates. It is necessary to limit the daily intake of table salt to 8g; the intake of free fluid should be about 1.5 liters. The caloric value of the diet should be 3100kcal with 5 meals a day.

It is allowed to consume almost all food products, but they must be served in boiled form, mashed. Steaming is recommended. It is permitted to eat low-fat varieties of fish and meat, even in baked form, but without a crisp.

It is not recommended to eat foods that linger in the stomach for a long time.

6.3 Diet N°3

6.3.1 Indications

Chronic intestinal diseases accompanied by hypomotor dyskinesia (persistent constipation).

6.3.2 Purpose

Recovery of impaired intestinal functions, stimulation of the regeneration of the mucous membrane, and restoration of impaired metabolism.

The diet is aimed at enhancing peristalsis, has the goal of emptying the intestines with the inclusion of mechanical, physical, and temperature stimuli in the diet. This diet is used for constipation, the cause of which is malnutrition, without pronounced signs of intestinal irritation.

6.3.3 General Characteristics

A physiologically complete diet with a normal protein, carbohydrate, and fat content, 30% of which is vegetable oil. The content of vitamins and minerals corresponds to the need for a healthy person.

6.3.4 Composition

Proteins 100g, fats 90-100g, carbohydrates 400g, sodium chloride 6-8g, calories 2500-2900kcal; retinol 2mg, thiamine 4mg, riboflavin 4mg, nicotinic acid 30mg, ascorbic acid 100mg; calcium 0.8g, phosphorus 1.2g, magnesium 0.5g, and iron 0.015g.

The food temperature is normal. Food is salted normally. The liquid is recommended to use in the amount of 1.2-1.5 liters.

It is recommended to eat at least 4-5 times a day, always at the same hours. Long breaks in time between separate meals are unacceptable.

When food products enter the upper gastrointestinal tract, this reflexively causes an increase in contractions of the lower intestine, which helps to speed up its emptying.

The nature of the culinary processing of food products also has a certain therapeutic value. In particular, when preparing salads and side dishes, carrots, radishes, and other vegetables should not be crushed very much; for this purpose, it is recommended to use a larger grater.

The diet includes dishes rich in plant fiber, but not irritating the gastrointestinal mucosa. It is recommended to include in the diet salads of fresh vegetables, herbs 100-150g 2-3 times a day, baked apples, stewed vegetables, diluted vegetable and fruit juices with the pulp. Food is prepared in any form (mainly in unmilled form, steamed or boiled in water).

In the absence of contraindications, it is preferable to take raw fruits and vegetables. Beets, carrots, tomatoes, leafy lettuce, zucchini, pumpkin, cauliflower, apples are especially recommended. Dried fruits (prunes, dried apricots, figs) are given in a soaked form and in dishes. White cabbage, green peas, young green beans are allowed with good tolerance. Greens parsley, dill, and celery can be added to various dishes and salads.

With constipation, people with inflammatory bowel diseases make up a diet, guided by the same principles, but in order to comply with the principle of sparing the mucous membrane from possible adverse effects of food, vegetables are used boiled.

6.3.5 Recommended Foods

- It is recommended to eat foods rich in fiber: vegetables and fruits, herbs, brown bread, sauerkraut, as well as carbonated drinks and hard-boiled eggs.

- Bread products - wheat bread from wholemeal flour, crispbread (soaked), rye bread, seeded and from wallpaper flour, bran, cereal, doctor's, yesterday's baking.

- Cookies and other dough products.

- Snacks - salads from fresh vegetables, vinaigrettes with vegetable oil; herring, red caviar. Salads, vinaigrettes with mayonnaise, jellyfish, and curd paste.

- Soups on weak fat-free meat, fish broth, vegetable broth, with pearl barley; cold soups; fruit and vegetable soups (beetroot soup, bovine, okroshka, sorrel soup, etc.). Borsch, beetroot soup, and cabbage soup from fresh cabbage.

- Meat, poultry, (products from beef, veal, poultry, lamb and pork), boiled fish of low-fat varieties, baked mainly with a piece.

- Dishes and side dishes from flour, cereals, legumes and pasta - crumbly and semi-viscous cereals, puddings, casseroles from cereals, pasta boiled and in the form of casseroles; buckwheat dishes are especially recommended. From legumes: green peas, beancurd.

- Fats - butter, olive oil, refined sunflower, and corn.

- Eggs and dishes from them - no more than one egg per day, if necessary, according to culinary indications only in dishes.

- Dishes and side dishes from vegetables and mushrooms - various types of vegetables and greens; non-acidic sauerkraut. Beetroot is especially recommended.

- Vegetables - beets, carrots, tomatoes, lettuce, cucumbers, zucchini, pumpkin, raw, boiled on a side dish and in the form of casseroles.

- Vegetables and fruits are allowed both raw and boiled and baked. Berries, fruits, and vegetables are recommended that stimulate intestinal function, but do not enhance fermentation and do not irritate the intestinal mucosa. Especially recommended: melons, plums, figs, apricots, prunes; sugar, jam, especially mountain ash, mousses, fruit, and sweets. Dried fruits soaked (dried apricots, prunes).

- Milk, dairy products, and dishes from them - milk (with tolerance - sweet), sour cream, cottage cheese, yogurt, one and two-day kefir, acidophilus milk, and cheeses.

- Sauces and spices - dairy, sour cream, vegetable broth, fruit, and berry gravy. Sauces on weak meat, fish stock.

- Drinks - tea is weak, tea with milk, coffee is not strong and natural with milk, fruit and berry juices, sweet. Juices are recommended cold.

- Vitamins - are given in the form of a decoction of rose hips, various sweet berry and fruit juices, raw vegetables and fruits, tomatoes, and raw carrot puree.

6.3.6 Excluded foods

- Hot dishes, jelly, and mashed cereals are limited.

- To reduce the negative impact on other organs of the digestive tract, which is especially important for combined pathology, they try to avoid vegetables rich in essential oils and fiber (onions, radishes, turnips, spinach, and peppers), mushrooms.

- Exclude foods rich in cholesterol, as well as fat breakdown products formed during frying.

- Bread from premium flour, butter bakery products.

- Fatty varieties of meat, fish, poultry; smoked meats, canned meat, and fish.

- Spicy and fatty sauces, horseradish, mustard, pepper, cocoa, strong tea, animals and cooking fats.

- Horseradish, pepper, mustard are excluded. Spices are excluded.

- Rice, semolina, and vermicelli.

- Legumes, radish, garlic, onions, and mushrooms.

- Kissel, blueberries, and quince.
- Chocolate, cream products, and cocoa.
- Rice and semolina are undesirable.
- Eggs and dishes from them - no more than one egg per day, if necessary, according to culinary indications only in dishes.
- The use of alcoholic beverages is prohibited.

6.3.7 Sample diet menu

6.3.7.1 Menu 1

- 1st breakfast. Oil. Cottage cheese with sour cream. Buckwheat porridge with butter. A glass of tea with milk.
- 2nd breakfast. Grated carrots with sour cream. A glass of broth of wild rose.
- Dinner. Vegetarian borsch with sour cream. Roasted meat with boiled potatoes and beets, sauerkraut. Fresh fruit compote (rhubarb).
- An afternoon snack. A glass of weak tea with crispbread and honey.
- Dinner. Cabbage rolls with carrots (vegetarian). Pie with dried fruits (prunes). A glass of weak tea.
- At night - fruit and berry compote.
- For the whole day: Coarse bread - 200g, rye bread - 200g, sugar - 50g.

6.3.7.2 Menu 2

- In the morning on an empty stomach: a glass of cold water with sugar, salt, jam or prune infusion, prunes, and cold lemonade.

- 1st breakfast: a glass of weak tea or coffee with milk, salad, vinaigrette or grated radish with carrots and sour cream or vegetable oil, 100g of cottage cheese or cheese, porridge made from oatmeal or Hercules flakes, 100g of rye bread or Borodino, "Health," 20g of oil.

- 2nd breakfast: raw apple, carrots, a glass of rosehip broth, 1 cup of kefir (yogurt), 100g of black bread, and 10g of butter.

- Lunch: sauerkraut cabbage soup, fruit or vegetable soup, okroshka, meat (fried or stewed), fish, chicken, side dishes of beets, cabbage, potatoes, zucchini, salad, fresh plum fruit compote, raisins, and fresh fruits.

- Dinner: fried fish with potatoes, cabbage, cucumber, buckwheat or barley porridge with butter, vegetable casserole, cottage cheese, stewed cabbage, vinaigrette, fruits, black bread and butter salad, grated radish with carrots and sour cream or kefir, weak tea with sugar, and jam.

- At night: kefir (1 cup), soaked prunes or mashed boiled beets, fruits, depending on the season.

6.4 Diet N°4

6.4.1 Indications

Acute and chronic intestinal diseases during profuse diarrhea and pronounced dyspeptic disorders, condition after bowel surgery.

6.4.2 Purpose

Maximum mechanical and chemical sparing of the intestine, a decrease in fermentation processes in it. With this diet, a restriction is made in the diet of chemical, mechanical, and thermal irritations to the intestines. The diet is indicated for bowel diseases occurring with diarrhea: dysentery, gastroenteritis during the exacerbation, and chronic colitis in the acute stage.

6.4.3 General characteristics

A diet with a normal amount of protein, limiting fats and carbohydrates to the lower limit of the norm. The purpose of this diet is to reduce the inflammatory changes in the intestinal mucosa by maximizing the mechanical and chemical ironing of the intestinal mucosa.

All dishes are boiled or steamed and wiped. Exclude foods and dishes that enhance the processes of fermentation and rotting in the intestines, in particular milk, sweets, legumes, coarse fiber (fresh vegetables, herbs, fruits, and berries), all dishes that stimulate bile secretion, secretion of the stomach and pancreas (sauces, spices, snacks). The diet should be fractionated to 5–6 times a day.

This diet option is physiologically inferior and monotonous; therefore, it is prescribed for 2–5 days, followed by transfer to table N°2 or N°5a.

6.4.4 Composition

Proteins 90g, fats 70g, carbohydrates 250g, sodium chloride 6g; calorie content 2000kcal; retinol 2mg, thiamine 4mg, riboflavin 4mg, ascorbic acid 100mg, nicotinic acid 30mg; calcium 0.8g, phosphorus 1.6g, magnesium 0.5g, iron 0.015g. Reduce the salt content in the diet to 6-8g per day. Free fluid 1.5 liters.

6.4.5 Recommended foods

- Bread in the form of crackers from 200g of wheat bread from premium flour; stale white bread.

- Soups on low-fat low-meat, fish broth with the addition of mucous decoctions of cereals (pearl barley, semolina, and rice), boiled and mashed meat, steam knives, meatballs, and egg flakes.

- Meat and poultry - low-fat and non-fatty varieties of beef, veal, turkey in the form of cutlets boiled on water, knlets, meatballs; boiled meat souffle.

- Fish - low-fat varieties of fresh fish, boiled in water or steam, in the form of meatballs, meatballs, or a piece.

- Dairy products - freshly prepared calcined cottage cheese or fresh mashed cottage cheese.

- Butter - fresh, added to dishes.

- Eggs - 1-2 soft-boiled or in the form of a steam omelet.

- Cereals - mashed cereals on the water (rice, oat, buckwheat).

- Vegetables - only in the form of decoctions added to soups.

- Drinks - tea, especially green, black coffee and cocoa on the water; diluted fruit juices from berries and fruits, except grapes, plums, apricots, jelly from blueberries, quinces, pears, decoctions of rose hips, dried blueberries, and black currants. A decoction of dried black currants, blueberries, and bird cherry.

- Rubbed raw apples.

6.4.6 Excluded foods

- Other than those listed above, bakery and flour products are excluded.

- Snacks are excluded.

- Soups with cereals and vegetables, strong and fatty broths.

- Fatty varieties of meat, fish, poultry; smoked meats, canned meat, and fish.

- Milk and dairy products.

- Millet, pearl barley, and barley groats.

- Legumes; natural vegetables, fruits, and berries.

- All sweets, coffee, and cocoa with milk, carbonated and cold drinks.

6.4.7 Variants and options

6.4.7.1 Diet N°4a

Diet N°4a is used for any bowel disease that occurs with a predominance of fermentation processes.

Diet N°4a sharply limits the content in the diet of all substances that irritate the intestines and enhance the fermentation processes in it. The calorie content of this table is 1600kcal, the composition of the diet: 120g of protein, 50g of fat, 140g of carbohydrates.

This diet option is physiologically inferior and monotonous; therefore, it is prescribed for 2–5 days, followed by transfer to table N°2 or N°5a.

6.4.7.1.1 An approximate one-day diet menu
(with a pronounced exacerbation of intestinal diseases, with diarrhea)

- 1st breakfast: protein steam omelet, semolina porridge on water, and tea.
- 2nd breakfast: calcified curd (100g).
- Lunch: meat soup puree, steamed meatballs, and blueberry jelly.
- Snack: broth of wild rose (1 cup).
- Dinner: aspic fish, boiled vermicelli, and tea.
- At night: kefir (1 glass).
- For the whole day: bread (crackers) - 200g, sugar - 30g, butter - 10g.

6.4.7.2 Diet N°4b

Diet N°4b is used in the period of exacerbation of chronic and acute intestinal diseases, with a combination of intestinal diseases with diseases of the pancreas, stomach, liver, and biliary tract.

This diet slightly limits the content of mechanical and chemical stimuli of the gastrointestinal receptor apparatus in the diet.

6.4.7.2.1 Purpose

Ensuring good nutrition with a moderate inflammatory process in the digestive tract and digestive disorders.

6.4.7.2.2 General characteristics

The diet is physiologically complete with a moderate restriction of mechanical and chemical irritants of the gastrointestinal tract, a moderate restriction of salt, except for products that enhance fermentation processes, as well as strong stimulants of gastric secretion and bile secretion. All dishes - boiled or steamed, mashed, mucous, served warm and hot. Dietary intake should be fractionated to 5-6 times a day.

Use products rich in tannin (blueberries, strong black tea, cocoa, natural red wines) containing simple carbohydrates to delay bowel movement. The daily intake should be divided to 6 meals a day. All products should be steamed or boiled; vegetables should come in mashed form, fruits - in the form of mashed potatoes.

6.4.7.2.3 Composition

Protein 100g, fat 100g, carbohydrates 350-400g; calorie content 2700-2900kcal; retinol 2mg, thiamine 4mg, riboflavin 4mg, nicotinic acid 30mg, ascorbic acid 100mg; calcium 0.8g, phosphorus 1.2g, magnesium 0.5g, and iron 0.015g. It is necessary to limit the amount of salt consumed to 8g per day. The amount of free fluid consumed should be 1.5 liters per day.

6.4.7.2.4 Recommended foods

- Wheat bread from the flour of the highest or first grade of yesterday's baking or dried. Total bakery products no more than 200g/day.

- Soups on weak meat, fish broth and vegetable broth with well-boiled and mashed cereals or finely chopped and well-boiled vegetables, as well as meatballs and dumplings.

- It allowed low-fat varieties of meat and fish (beef, veal, rabbit, chicken, pike perch, bream, cod, and perch) in the form of boiled meatballs, dumplings, soufflé (with good tolerance in the form of a whole piece).

- Various cereals in the form of well-boiled cereals, on water or with the addition of 1/3 of milk.

- Vegetables - potatoes, carrots, boiled and mashed cauliflower; ripe fruits and sweet varieties of berries without a peel. With good tolerance, ripe tomatoes are allowed (up to 100g/day).

- Dairy products - milk, cream, sour cream, added to the dish, kefir, acidophilus, yogurt, and freshly prepared cottage cheese.

- Unsalted butter is added to ready meals or in its natural form with bread up to 15g per reception.

- Soft-boiled eggs can be eaten (up to 2 eggs per day) or in the form of additives to dishes, egg white omelets, meringues, and snowballs.

- In contrast to diet N°4 and N°4a, snacks are allowed (mild cheese, doctor's sausage, pasta, veal, soaked herring, jellied meat, jellied tongue) and sauces (on meat, vegetable and fishy weak broths with dill, parsley leaves, milk sauce bechamel with a small amount of sour cream, fruit sauces, cinnamon can be used).

- As sources of vitamins use jelly, mousse, mashed compotes from sweet berries and fruits (except melons, watermelons, apricots, and plums), baked apples, raw berries (strawberries, raspberries up to 100g), mashed peeled ripe sweet apples and pears. Fruit juices diluted 1:1 with water are allowed. Their intake begins with 50ml, gradually increasing to 100-150ml per day.

- Drinks - tea, coffee, and cocoa in water or milk.

6.4.7.2.5 Excluded foods

- From the daily diet, it is necessary to exclude all products that stimulate bile secretion. The secretory activity of the stomach and pancreas enhances putrefactive and fermentation processes in the intestine.

- Other than those listed above, bakery and flour products are excluded.

- Soups with cereals and vegetables, strong and fatty broths are excluded.

- Fatty varieties of meat, fish, poultry, smoked meats, canned meat, and fish.

- Millet, pearl barley, and barley groats.

- Legumes; natural vegetables, fruits, and berries.

- All sweets, coffee, and cocoa with milk, carbonated and cold drinks.

6.4.7.2.6 Approximate one-day diet menu (for patients with acute or chronic intestinal diseases in the phase of subsiding exacerbation)

- 1st breakfast: boiled fish, mashed potatoes, mashed rice porridge, and tea.

- 2nd breakfast: calcified curd (100g).

- Lunch: cheese (30g), pearl barley soup with meat broth with mashed carrots, meatloaf with mashed buckwheat porridge, and apple jelly.

- Snack: broth of wild rose (1/2 cup) and protein omelet.

- Dinner: boiled tongue with mashed carrots and calcified curd.

- At night: kefir (1 glass).

- For the whole day: white bread - 300g, sugar - 50g, butter - 10g, fruits, berries - 300g.

6.4.7.3 Diet N°4c

Diet N°4c is prescribed during the recovery period after acute intestinal diseases as a transitional table to general nutrition, as well as during the period of remission of intestinal diseases, with a combination of intestinal diseases with diseases of the pancreas, stomach, liver and biliary tract.

Diet N°4c, in comparison with diet N°4b, is more diverse and less sparing; therefore, it is prescribed after a 2-4-week use of diet N°4b.

6.4.7.3.1 Purpose

Providing proper nutrition and compensating digestion in chronic intestinal diseases in remission, in acute intestinal diseases in recovery.

6.4.7.3.2 General characteristics

Diet N°4c is physiologically complete, with normal content of proteins, fats, and carbohydrates, with a certain restriction of salt, chemical irritants, except for foods and dishes that enhance the processes of fermentation and decay in the intestines. All dishes are cooked in water or steam, and baked in the oven; food is mostly unground. The dietary intake should be fractionated to 6 times a day.

6.4.7.3.3 Composition

Proteins 100-110g, fats 90-100g, carbohydrates 400-450g; calorie content 2900-3140kcal; retinol 2mg, thiamine 4mg, riboflavin 4mg, nicotinic acid 30mg, ascorbic acid 100mg; calcium 1.2g, phosphorus 1.6g, magnesium 0.5g, iron 0.015g. It is necessary to limit the amount of salt consumed to 8g per day. The amount of freely consumed fluid should be 1.5 liters per day.

6.4.7.3.4 Recommended foods

- Wheat bread from the flour of the highest or first grade of yesterday's baking or dried.

- Soups on weak meat, fish broth and vegetable broth with well-boiled and mashed cereals or finely chopped and well-boiled vegetables, as well as meatballs and dumplings.

- Meat and poultry - meat, chicken, turkey - chopped, steamed, or boiled.

- Fish - low-fat varieties by piece, chopped, from boiled or steam; individual dishes are baked, without a rough crust.

- Loose porridge (except for millet and pearl barley) on water, on meat broth, with the addition of milk or a third part of 10% cream, zraza, dumplings, pancakes, boiled vermicelli, finely chopped pasta, milk noodles in the form of side dishes, casseroles, puddings are allowed.

- Dairy products - milk, cream, sour cream, added to the dish, kefir, acidophilus, yogurt, and freshly prepared cottage cheese.

- Butter is added to the finished dishes and is given in its natural form (no more than 10g per 1 reception).

- Eggs - 1-2 eggs per day in the form of omelet or soft-boiled.

- Sauces on weak meat, fish broth, and dairy.

- Vegetables - potatoes, carrots, boiled and mashed cauliflower; ripe fruits and sweet varieties of berries without a peel. With good tolerance, the addition of white cabbage, green peas, young beans, and beets to soups is allowed. Young finely chopped greens, tangerines, and oranges are introduced into the diet.

- Drinks - tea, coffee, cocoa in water or milk. The amount of raw sweet fruits and berries (apples, pears, strawberries) is increased to 200g/day. Showing fruit juices (except grape), berry, vegetable (except cabbage), diluted 1/3 with water.

- Marmalade, candy, marshmallows, and sugar are allowed.

6.4.7.3.5 Excluded foods

- Other than those listed above, bakery and flour products are excluded.
- Soups with cereals and vegetables, strong and fatty broths.
- Fatty varieties of meat, fish, poultry, smoked meats, canned meat, and fish.
- Legumes; natural vegetables, fruits, and berries.
- Coffee and cocoa, carbonated and cold drinks.

6.4.7.3.6 Approximate diet menu (for patients with acute or chronic intestinal diseases that occur with diarrhea during the recovery period or in the remission phase)

- 1st breakfast: milk rice porridge, steam protein omelet (2 eggs), and tea with milk.
- 2nd breakfast: calcified curd (150g).
- Lunch: soup on meat broth with cauliflower, boiled meat with boiled rice, and fresh apples.
- Snack: boiled meat, rosehip broth (200g).
- Dinner: baked curd pudding, meat steamroll with stewed carrots and green peas, tea with milk, and fresh fruits (or berries).
- At night: kefir (1 glass).
- For the whole day: white bread - 300g, sugar - 40g, butter - 10g.

6.4.7.4 Diet N°4d (gluten-free diet)

A special variant of diet N°4 is diet N°4d, intended for patients with gluten enteropathy, in which the body loses its ability to digest gluten (an integral part of cereal proteins) due to the absence of specific peptidase in the epithelium of the intestinal mucosa, as a result of which the gliadin is part of gluten-free.

Diet N°4d contains an increased amount of proteins, the physiological norm of fat, and is enriched with vitamins and calcium salts. Foods are boiled or steamed.

6.4.7.4.1 Composition

Protein 120g, fat 100g, carbohydrates 400-450g, sodium chloride 8g; calorie content 2980 - 3180kcal.

6.4.7.4.2 Dietary strategies for celiac disease (celiac enteropathy)

In extremely severe cases of dystrophy, treatment for celiac disease begins with parenteral nutrition in the intensive care unit. See parenteral nutrition.

The minimum requirement of the body for the protein needed by the body to avoid the destruction of its own structural proteins is 0.6-0.9g/kg per day.

Parenteral nutrition begins with the lower limit of daily protein requirements (0.6g/kg), given the poor tolerance of the protein with severe depletion.

The next day, the amount of protein is prescribed at the rate of 1g/kg, gradually increases to 2-3g/kg. Basically, the protein requirement for parenteral nutrition is made up of special amino acid mixtures.

As diarrhea is eliminated and the necessary amount of fluid is replenished, the dose of protein increases to 4g/kg, while the amount of protein introduced with food increases, and in the form of amino acid preparations, it decreases.

Another component of therapy for severe conditions is fat emulsions, administered separately from other solutions (3-4 times). When the condition improves, fats are administered as nutrition, using special preparations for enteral nutrition.

The need for parenteral carbohydrate nutrition is met by the intravenous administration of glucose and fructose in 5, 10, and 20% solutions under the control of blood sugar levels.

In the first 2-3 days of parenteral nutrition, patients may have weight loss due to the disappearance of edema, stabilization occurs in the next 2-3 days, and by the end of the week, the patient's body weight begins to increase. Lethargy and unwillingness to move will disappear after 3-4 days. By the end of the second week, patients get up and move independently. Vomiting stops from the first day of treatment; the number of bowel movements decreases to 3 times a day.

The prognosis for further adherence to the gluten-free diet is favorable. It is believed that a strict gluten-free diet should be carried out for at least 8-10 months. After that, it is allowed to introduce products containing gluten carefully. But if at the same time, the stool becomes more frequent again, one should immediately return to the previous diet.

6.4.7.4.3 General nutritional guidelines

- For children, food should be age-appropriate, rubbed (sparing). The volumes of one serving are small, and the number of feedings can be increased. The child can drink at will, without restrictions.

- Culinary processing of products in the initial period of treatment - stewing, cooking, and a little more than usual. Pass the products through a meat grinder, rub, or rub through a sieve. Peel vegetables and fruits. It is better to refuse grapes and grape juice at the beginning of treatment, since the berries have a hard skin, and juice can cause fermentation in the intestines and bloat.

- The first few months of the diet are not recommended to include mushrooms, legumes, nuts, raw cabbage, and apples, as they contain coarse fiber, which can slow down intestinal recovery. Limit garlic, onions, and spices.

- Whole milk should be limited. This restriction is especially true for factory milk, in which flour can often be added.

- Domestic milk and non-industrial dairy products can be used in the absence of lactase deficiency.

- Sweets do not limit. Simple carbohydrates will partially make up for metabolic disorders, and improve brain nutrition. As recovery is reached, the need for sweets will decrease.

The main sources of food ingredients:

- Protein: meat, fish, natural dairy products, and eggs.

- Fat: vegetable oil, fat found in meat, homemade milk, and fish.

- Carbohydrates: rice, corn, buckwheat (limited), potato starch, rice, corn, vegetables, fruits, jam, honey, and sugar.

- Biological products (bifidumbacterin, lactobacterin), constantly, 5-10 doses daily, on an empty stomach or at bedtime 2 hours after eating.

- Sea buckthorn oil and honey. 1-2 tsp. daily, but not together.

6.4.7.4.4 Criteria for the effectiveness of diet therapy for celiac disease

The exclusion of gluten-containing foods from the diet leads to the rapid disappearance of symptoms, and then normalization of all biochemical parameters. The first sign of recovery is the elimination of rapid and profuse stools. Then there is an increase in body weight and the disappearance of all symptoms of insufficiency in the body. Osteoporosis is most slowly eliminated; therefore, in addition to diet therapy, it is necessary to take calcium and vitamin D preparations. Over the course of 3–8 months of treatment, health, working capacity, and mood improve.

6.4.7.4.5 Dosage forms approved for celiac disease

- All those dosage forms that do not contain wheat starch.

- It is better to use only ampoule preparations, using them as tablets, dissolving in water; candles and transparent gelatin capsules.

- In tablets, only activated charcoal can be taken - it contains potato starch.

6.4.7.4.6 Recommended foods

- Children under 3-4 months are only allowed breast milk.

- Adults include gluten-free foods - rice, corn, starch, soy, hazelnuts, vegetables, and fruits.

- Corn and rice flour, potatoes, meat, and fish are allowed.

- Buckwheat porridge is indicated in limited quantities.

- Vegetable oil and oil made from pure cow cream.

- Fresh sour cream, fresh cream (weighted, non-industrial).

- Cottage cheese, cheeses, and fermented milk products made from draft milk at home.

- Meat (all varieties), eggs, fish, canned fish in its own juice, and oil.

- Caviar.

- All kinds of fruits in kind (except bananas and dates), all vegetables.

- Sugar, honey, whole coffee beans (to be ground), and loose tea.

- Homemade canned food (meat, jam).

- Industrial canned food (sprats, seaweed, and canned corn).

6.4.7.4.7 Excluded foods

Prohibited Products

- Children are contraindicated in the introduction of mixtures with decoctions of oats, barley, and wheat. For older children, bread, cookies, semolina, oatmeal, and crackers are excluded.

- Wheat, rye, barley, oats, as well as all products containing them, are completely excluded from nutrition. (From millet, groats are made, from oats - oat groats (Hercules), from wheat - semolina and wheat groats, wheat flour. From barley - pearl barley and barley groats, from rye - rye flour.)

- Milk mixtures with oat and wheat broths and flour are forbidden, sour-milk mixtures with oat and wheat broths and flour.

- Canned meat, homogenized canned meat containing flour, and ham. All products (semi-finished products, meatballs, and cheesecakes), breaded in breadcrumbs or with the addition of bread, and sausages.

- Breaded fish, canned fish in which flour is added.

- Vegetables and canned vegetables, which is added wheat or oat flour, and barley.

- Products made from wheat, barley, biscuits, cookies, and gingerbread cookies.

- Canned fruit compotes.

- All confectionery, sweets, caramel, dragees, and chocolate. All home and industrial baked products from wheat, rye, and buckwheat flour (bread, rolls, dryers, crackers, cakes, and pastries).

- Cornflakes.

- Sauces, mustard.

- Bouillon cubes.

- Beer, vodka.

- Carbonated drinks.

- Bananas, dates.

Products not recommended

- Air bread, corn sticks, cereal, and chips.

- Ice cream, yogurts, all kinds of curd cakes, curd and curd mass, packaged cottage cheese, powdered or condensed milk, cream, margarine, and industrial butter, cheeses, and mayonnaise.

- Ketchup, tomato paste.

- Cocoa, Pepsi-Cola, Coca-Cola, instant coffee, and granulated tea. Marshmallows, jams, pastille, Turkish delight, and halva.

- All tablet forms of drugs, dragees, opaque capsules, syrups, and peas.

- Chewing gums and toothpaste.

- Cosmetics (lipstick and mascara).

6.4.7.4.8 Gluten-free sample diet menu

Menu for the week for adults

Monday

- First breakfast: rice porridge on the water, grated cheese, and tea.

- Second breakfast: apple (mashed potatoes).

- Lunch: vegetarian soup, meat with mashed potatoes on a vegetable broth, and compote.
- Snack: apple (mashed potatoes).
- Dinner: meat with mashed potatoes on a vegetable broth and tea.

Tuesday

- First breakfast: buckwheat porridge on the water, grated cheese, and tea.
- Second breakfast: apple (mashed potatoes).
- Lunch: vegetarian potato soup, mashed potatoes with mashed potatoes, and compote.
- Snack: orange.
- Dinner: rice porridge on the water, soft-boiled egg, and tea.

Wednesday

- First breakfast: buckwheat porridge on the water, scrambled eggs without milk, and tea.
- Second breakfast: homemade cottage cheese.

- Lunch: vegetarian soup, meat with mashed potatoes on a vegetable broth, and compote.

- Snack: orange or apple.

- Dinner: grated rice porridge on water, soft-boiled egg, and tea.

Thursday

- First breakfast: rice porridge on the water and tea.

- Second breakfast: homemade cottage cheese.

- Lunch: vegetarian soup, meat with mashed potatoes on a vegetable broth, and compote.

- Snack: apple (mashed potatoes).

- Dinner: buckwheat porridge on the water mashed, soft-boiled egg, and tea.

Friday

- First breakfast: buckwheat porridge on the water, soft-boiled egg, and tea.

- Second breakfast: apple (mashed potatoes).

- Lunch: vegetarian potato soup, meat with mashed potatoes on a vegetable broth, and compote.
- Snack: apple (mashed potatoes).
- Dinner: rice porridge on the water, meat, and tea.

Saturday

- First breakfast: rice porridge on the water, grated cheese, and tea.
- Second breakfast: apple (mashed potatoes).
- Lunch: vegetarian soup, meat with mashed potatoes on a vegetable broth, and compote.
- Snack: apple (mashed potatoes).
- Dinner: meat with mashed potatoes on a vegetable broth and tea.

Sunday

- First breakfast: buckwheat porridge on the water, grated cheese, and tea.
- Second breakfast: homemade cottage cheese.

- Lunch: vegetarian soup, meat puree with mashed potatoes on a vegetable broth, and compote.

- Snack: apple.

- Dinner: rice porridge on the water, soft-boiled egg, and tea.

6.4.7.4.9 Gluten-free recipes

- **Cottage cheese**

Requires: 200 g of cottage cheese, sour milk, 1 egg, 1 tbsp. 1 gluten-free butter or cream, 1 tsp. soda, and salt.

Cooking: pour cottage cheese with sour milk 3 cm above the level of cottage cheese, boil for 10 minutes over low heat, put in a colander, let drain. Mix thoroughly with egg, cream, soda (salt to taste), cook for 5 minutes in a boiling water bath with stirring. Tamp in a bowl greased with vegetable oil, allow to cool.

- **Gluten-free butter**

Requires: heavy cream.

Cooking: Let the cream stand at room temperature for 30-40 minutes. Beat until stratified into oil and whey. Add to baked goods and ready meals.

- **Homemade cottage cheese**

Requires: 2 liters of milk, 3-4 tbsp. of fermented milk product.

Cooking: add the starter to milk, leave at room temperature for a day, warm over low heat in the oven. Cool, recline on a sieve. Serum can be used for making pancakes, okroshka, and drinking.

- **Hominy**

Requires: 1 cup corn grits, 4 cups milk (water), 50g gluten-free oil, and salt.

Cooking: Boil milk with butter (25g), add salt and corn grits and cook. Stir until the porridge begins to lag behind the walls of the pan. Stir in hot mamalyga with melted gluten-free oil (25g) before removing from heat. Cut the cold mamalyga into thin slices, dip in beaten eggs or roll in cornmeal, fry in oil, and serve with meat dishes.

- **Cheese pancakes made from cornmeal**

Requires: 0.5kg of cottage cheese, 1 egg, 3 tbsp. of sugar, cornmeal, raisins by weight or apples.

Cooking: beat eggs with sugar, put cottage cheese, mix, add flour until a stable dough is added, add raisins (apples), form cottage cheese pancakes, bake over medium heat until cooked.

- **Mayonnaise**

Requires: 2 yolks, salt, sugar, 0.5 cups of vegetable oil, 1 tsp. of vinegar.

Cooking: mix the ingredients, beat with a mixer.

- **Whipped cream with sugar**

    Requires: 1 cup cream, 2-3 tsp. of sahara.

    Cooking: cool the cream, add sugar, beat.

- **Ice cream**

    Requires: 700ml of milk, 300ml of homemade cream, 3 yolks, 150g of sugar, and 5g of gelatin.

    Cooking: soak gelatin for 30 minutes in a small amount of milk. Boil all milk, cool to 60 °C, add cream, put in a water bath. Beat egg yolks with sugar, add to milk, keep in a water bath for 15 minutes, stirring and not boiling. Introduce gelatin, beat, and strain. Cool at room temperature, refrigerate for 4-5 hours. Beat with a mixer, put in the freezer for 30-40 minutes. Beat again. Store in a freezer, divided into portions. Ice cream can only be made with cream, with milk alone - the ratio can be different.

- **Meat in sour cream**

    Requires: 500g of meat, 250g of sour cream, and garlic (2-3 cloves).

    Cooking: boil the meat, cool, and chop finely. Grate a few cloves of garlic in sour cream, ground black pepper to taste. Then mix.

- **Hepatic pancakes**

    Requires: 300g of liver, 0.5 cups of milk, 1 potato tuber, 1 egg, 1 onion, and cornmeal.

Cooking: pass the liver through a meat grinder, fry the onions in vegetable oil, and grate potatoes on a coarse grater. To mix, add salt and flour. Bake in vegetable oil.

- **Fritters with onions**

Requires: 2-3 tbsp. l homemade cottage cheese, 1 egg, 1 clove of garlic, 2-3 tbsp. l cornmeal, salt, red pepper, and soda.

Cooking: grind the cottage cheese with the egg, chop the onion, garlic, and mix everything. Bake in vegetable oil, close the pan with a lid.

- **Carrot cake**

Requires: 2 cups of grated carrots on a fine grater, 1 cup of granulated sugar, 2 eggs, 2 cups of cornmeal, 1 tsp. soda.

Cooking: mix carrots with sugar and leave for 30 minutes. Beat eggs, mix everything. Knead the dough. Divide into 2-3 parts (cakes). Bake on tracing paper, spreading cakes with jam.

- **Meatloaf with buckwheat porridge and mushrooms**

Requires: 100g of meat, 60g of buckwheat, 1-2 dried mushrooms, 1 onion, 1 tbsp. l vegetable oil, 1 tbsp. l cornmeal, 1 egg, salt, and pepper.

Cooking: carefully sort through the cereals, leaving only whole grains, rinse several times in cold water. Grind the meat, mix with 1/2 egg. Soak the mushrooms, cook, and chop finely. Finely chop the onion, spasser. Buckwheat to cook. Connect everything. Make a roll, grease the surface with sour cream or milk with the rest of the egg. Bake on low heat.

- **Omelet with buckwheat porridge**

Requires: 2 eggs, 1 tbsp. of vegetable oil, 100g buckwheat porridge, 1/4 cup milk.

Cooking: Beat the eggs with a mixer and pour it into a hot pan. In the middle of the omelet, put buckwheat porridge, wrap the edges of the omelet in the form of a pie, and put on a plate. Sprinkle with dill and serve.

- **Grated pie**

Required: for the test: 200g of vegetable oil, 300g of cornmeal, 60g of sugar, 2 yolks, 1/2 tsp. soda; for a layer: 3 egg whites, 100g of sugar, 100g of ground walnuts, 150g of jam.

Cooking: mix flour with soda, add vegetable oil, sugar, and yolks. Knead the dough, keep it for 2 hours in the refrigerator. For a layer, beat the whites in a strong foam, add nuts and sugar. On a baking sheet, grate half the dough on a coarse grater, put the protein mixture, grate the second half of the dough on top. Oven at a temperature of 180 °C for 30 minutes.

- **King's pie**

Requires: 5 eggs, 1 tsp. of salt, 200g of mineral water, 200g of refined sunflower oil, 300g of cornmeal, soda, 200g of finely chopped meat, 1 pickled cucumber, and 1 bell pepper.

Cooking: mix everything and bake.

- **Lazy meat pie**

    Requires: 300g of minced meat, 1 onion, 4 eggs, soda, 5 tbsp. l corn flour, 5 tbsp. of a mixture of corn starch and rice flour, 200ml of mineral water.

    Cooking: mix everything, pour into a greased form, and bake.

- **Cookies**

    Requires: 8 tbsp. of sugar, 8 tbsp. of vegetable oil, 1/2 tsp. of soda, and cornmeal.

    Cooking: mix everything, add enough cornmeal to make a thick dough. Form a cookie with a spoon and put it on a baking sheet. Allow to stand for 20 minutes, bake in a hot oven.

- **Okroshka**

    Requires: 50g of boiled meat, 50g of boiled tongue, 60g of cucumbers, 30g of green onions, 1/4 eggs, 1 tbsp. of sour cream, 1 tsp. of sugar, 350ml of whey, and salt.

    Cooking: finely chop everything, mix with whey, and allow to cool. Before serving, put dill and sour cream.

- **Cornmeal fritters**

    Requires: 1 egg, 250g of draft milk, 3 tsp. of sugar, 0.3 tsp soda, and cornmeal.

    Cooking: beat eggs with sugar, add milk, mix soda with cornflour. Add flour in portions to make a thick dough, like sour cream. Bake over medium heat under a lid.

- **Cornmeal cutlets**

    Requires: 0.5kg of minced chicken, 1 egg, 5 tbsp. of cornmeal, and 1 onion.

    Cooking: chop onion, mix with egg and minced meat, add flour, mix, fry on low heat for at least 20 minutes on each side.

- **Corn roll**

    Requires: 1 cup of corn grits, 3 cups of water, 3 tbsp. of stewed cabbage, 1 tbsp. of potato starch, minced meat with onion and egg for the filling.

    Cooking: cook cereals, mix with stewed cabbage and starch, put on a clean towel moistened with water. Put the minced meat in the middle and wrap it in the form of a roll. Grease with egg and bake for 30 minutes.

- **Marmalade**

    Requires: 1kg of apples, 600g of sugar, 150g of sour cream, 200g of cornmeal, 1 tsp. of soda.

    Cooking: bake apples in the oven, rub through a sieve, mix with sugar, boil over low heat, stirring until thickened. Pour on a sheet of parchment, sprinkled with icing sugar, smooth, and cool.

- **Puff pastry on sour cream**

    Requires: for the test: 400g of sour cream, 2 eggs, 200g of cornmeal, 1 tsp. of soda; for cream: 250g of sour cream, 1/2 cup of sugar.

Cooking: beat eggs, add sour cream in portions. Put soda. Pour cornmeal in parts until sour cream is thick. Pour the dough into two wide and low forms, greased with vegetable oil, let it stand for 15-20 minutes, bake over medium heat. Cool the cakes, cut, grease with jam, sour cream, whipped with sugar. Keep refrigerated.

- **Meringue**

Requires: protein; 2 eggs, 1 cup of sugar.

Cooking: beat the proteins in a strong foam, adding sugar (beat until the mass ceases to spread). Put on a baking sheet with a teaspoon, put in a hot oven and bake on low heat for 1-1.5 hours without opening the oven.

- **Biscuit**

Requires: 1.5 cups of cornmeal, 1 cup of sugar, and 7 eggs.

Cooking: beat eggs, gradually adding sugar. Pour in flour. Layout the dough in forms coated with tracing paper, filling to 0.7 heights, bake for 40–45 minutes.

- **Pumpkin Pudding**

Requires: 150g of pumpkin, 60g of corn, 1 egg, 100ml of milk, 1 tsp. of sugar, vegetable oil.

Cooking: peel, chop, boil the pumpkin in half the milk and cook the corn grits in the rest of the milk. Wipe the pumpkin, combine everything, and bake.

6.5 Diet N°5

6.5.1 Indications

Chronic hepatitis of a progressive but benign course with signs of mild functional liver failure, chronic cholecystitis, gallstone disease, and acute hepatitis during the recovery period. The diet is also used for chronic colitis with a tendency to constipation, chronic gastritis without sharp violations, and chronic pancreatitis in remission.

6.5.2 Purpose

Providing the physiological needs of the body in nutrients and energy, restoring the impaired functions of the liver and biliary tract, mechanical and biochemical sparing of the stomach and intestines, which, as a rule, are involved in the pathological process. It carries out camping and unloading of fat and cholesterol metabolism, as well as stimulation of normal bowel activity.

Diet N°5 can be used for a long time; for 1.5-2 years, it should be expanded only on the recommendation of a doctor. During periods of exacerbation of liver diseases, it is recommended that the patient be transferred to a more sparing diet N°5a.

6.5.3 General Characteristics

Physiologically normal content of proteins and carbohydrates while limiting refractory fats, nitrogenous extractives, and cholesterol. All dishes are cooked boiled or steamed and baked in the oven. Wipe only sinewy meat and fiber-rich vegetables. Flour and vegetables do not make a passer. The temperature of the prepared dishes is 20–52 °C.

6.5.4 Composition

Proteins 100g, fats 90g (of which 1/3 are vegetable), carbohydrates 300-350g (of which simple carbohydrates 50-60g); calorie content 2800-3000kcal; retinol 0.5mg, carotene 10.5mg, thiamine 2mg, riboflavin 4mg, nicotinic acid 20mg, ascorbic acid 200mg; sodium 4g, potassium 4.5g, calcium 1.2g, phosphorus 1.6g, magnesium 0.5g, iron 0.015g. The daily intake of sodium chloride is 6-10g, free fluid - up to 2 liters. Compliance with the principle of frequent and fractional nutrition - meals every 3-4 hours in small portions.

6.5.5 Recommended foods

- Wheat bread from flour I and II grade, rye from seeded peeled flour, and yesterday's baking. Non-edible baking products can be added with boiled meat and fish, cottage cheese, apples, and dry biscuit.

- Vegetable and cereal soups on a vegetable broth, dairy with pasta, fruit, vegetarian borscht and cabbage soup; flour and vegetables for dressing are not fried, but dried; meat, fish and mushroom broths are excluded.

- Meat and poultry - low-fat beef, veal, pork, rabbit, chicken in boiled or baked form after boiling. They use meat, poultry without skin and fish of non-greasy varieties boiled, baked after boiling, in a piece or chopped. Doctoral, dairy and diabetic sausages, non-fat low-fat ham, dairy sausages, herring soaked in milk, jellied fish (after boiling) are allowed; fish stuffed with vegetables; seafood salads.

- Low-fat dairy products - milk, kefir, acidophilus, and yogurt. Bold curd up to 20% fat in its natural form and the form of casseroles, puddings, lazy dumplings, yogurt, and buttermilk. Sour cream is used only as a seasoning for dishes.

- Eggs are recommended in the form of omelets or soft-boiled, hard-boiled eggs, and fried eggs are desirable to exclude.

- Cereals - any dishes from cereals.

- Various vegetables in boiled, baked and stewed form; spinach, sorrel, radish, radish, garlic, and mushrooms are excluded.

- From sauces, sour cream, milk, vegetable, sweet vegetable gravy are shown, from spices - dill, parsley, and cinnamon.

- Appetizers - fresh vegetable salad with vegetable oil, fruit salads, and vinaigrettes. Fruits, non-acidic berries, compotes, and jelly.

- Sweets - meringues, snowballs, marmalade, not chocolates, honey, and jam are allowed. Sugar is partially replaced by xylitol or sorbitol.

- Drinks - tea, coffee with milk, fruit, berry and vegetable juices.

6.5.6 Excluded Foods

- Excluded from the menu are foods rich in extractive substances, oxalic acid, and essential oils that stimulate the secretory activity of the stomach and pancreas.

- Meat, fish, and mushroom broths; okroshka and salted cabbage soup are excluded.

- Fatty varieties of meat and fish, liver, kidneys, brains, smoked meats, salted fish, caviar, most sausages, and canned foods are undesirable.

- Excluded pork, beef, and lamb; cooking fats.

- Goose, duck, liver, kidneys, brains, smoked meats, sausages, canned meat, and fish are excluded; fatty varieties of meat, poultry, and fish.

- Hard-boiled and fried eggs are excluded.

- Fresh bread is excluded. Puff pastry and pastry, pastries, cakes, and fried pastries remain prohibited.

- Excludes cream, milk 6% fat.

- Legumes, sorrel, radishes, green onions, garlic, mushrooms, and pickled vegetables.

- Extreme caution should be taken with hot spices: horseradish, mustard, pepper, and ketchup.

- Chocolate, cream products, black coffee, and cocoa are excluded.

6.5.7 Sample Diet Menu for One Day

Menu 1:

- First breakfast. Curd pudding - 150g. Oatmeal - 150g. Tea with milk - 1 cup.

- Lunch. Raw carrots, fruits - 150g. Tea with lemon - 1 cup.

- Dinner. Vegetarian potato soup with sour cream - 1 plate. Boiled meat baked in white milk sauce - 125g. Zucchini stewed in sour cream - 200g. Kissel from apple juice - 200g.

- An afternoon snack. Rosehip broth - 1 cup. Cracker.

- Dinner. Boiled fish - 100g. Mashed potatoes - 200g. Tea with lemon - 1 cup.

- For the whole day: white bread - 200g, rye bread - 200g, sugar - 50-70g.

Menu 2:

- First breakfast. Protein omelet from 2 proteins - 100g. Tea with milk - 1 cup.

- Lunch. Baked apples - 100g

- Dinner. Rice soup with mashed vegetables ½ serving. Boiled chickens in white sauce - 115g. Buckwheat porridge, mashed - 150g. Milk jelly - 125g.

- An afternoon snack. Rusks with sugar. Rosehipbroth - 1 cup.

- Dinner. Boiled fish - 85g. Mashed potato - 150g. Tea with milk - 1 cup.

- Before bedtime. Fruit jelly - 1 glass.

- For the whole day: White bread - 200g, rye bread - 200g, sugar - 50-70g.

6.5.8 Variants and options

Various variants of the basic diet N°5 have been developed. The purpose of diet options N°5 are determined by the patient's condition and depends on the severity of the patient's condition and the presence of concomitant diseases.

6.5.8.1 Diet N°5a

6.5.8.1.1 Indications

Acute hepatitis, acute cholecystitis, cholangitis, exacerbation of chronic hepatitis and cholecystitis at the stage of exacerbation of diseases of the liver and biliary tract, with their combination with colitis and gastritis, and chronic colitis.

6.5.8.1.2 Purpose

Providing good nutrition in conditions of pronounced inflammatory changes in the liver and bile ducts, maximizing the tenderness of the affected organs, normalizing the functional state of the liver and other digestive organs. This table is based on the principles of table N°5 and the exclusion of mechanical irritations of the stomach and intestines.

6.5.8.1.3 General Characteristics

Physiologically complete, mechanically, biochemically, and thermally sparing. A diet with a normal protein and carbohydrate content, with some limitation of fat and salt. In order to detoxify the body for the first time (up to 3-5 days), increase the intake of free fluid; with fluid retention in the body, sodium chloride is limited to 3g/day.

Excluded are foods containing coarse fiber. All dishes are boiled, steamed, or mashed; stewing, sautéing, and roasting are excluded. The temperature of the prepared dishes is 20–52 °C. Compliance with the principle of frequent and fractional nutrition - meals every 3-4 hours (5-6 times a day) in small portions.

Diet N°5a is prescribed for 1.5-2 weeks, and then gradually, the patient is transferred to diet N°5. Diet N°5a is also transitional after diet N°4.

6.5.8.1.4 Composition

Proteins 80-100g, fats 70-80g, carbohydrates 350-400g; calorie content 2350 - 2700kcal; retinol 0.4mg, carotene 11.6mg, thiamine 1.3mg, riboflavin 2mg, nicotinic acid 16mg, ascorbic acid 100mg; sodium 3g, potassium 3.4g, calcium 0.8g, magnesium 0.4g, phosphorus 1.4g, iron 0.040g. The daily intake of sodium chloride is 6-10g, free liquid - up to 2-2.5l.

6.5.8.1.5 Recommended foods

- Bread and bakery products: white bread, dried; dry, inedible cookies.

- Soups: vegetarian, dairy, with mashed vegetables and cereals, milk soups in half with water.

- Meat, fish, and poultry dishes: chopped steam products (souffle, knelles, and meatballs). Chicken without skin and fish (low-fat varieties) in boiled form is allowed in pieces.

- Dishes and side dishes from vegetables: potatoes, carrots, beets, pumpkin, zucchini, cauliflower - in the form of mashed potatoes and steam soufflé; raw grated vegetables.

- Dishes from cereals, legumes, and pasta: liquid mashed and viscous cereals in milk from oat, buckwheat, rice, and semolina; mashed steam puddings; boiled vermicelli.

- Dishes from eggs: protein steam omelets.

- Sweet dishes, fruits, berries: mashed potatoes, juices, jelly, mashed compotes, mousse, sambuca, soufflé from sweet varieties of berries and fruits; baked apples.

- Milk and dairy products: milk, kefir, yogurt, acidophilus, fermented baked milk, mild cheese, sour cottage cheese and puddings from it.

- Sauces: on vegetable and cereal broths, milk, and fruit. Only fat-free white flour is used.

- Fruits: berries are ripe, soft, sweet in raw and mashed form.
- Drinks: tea, tea with milk, and rosehip broth.
- Fats: butter and vegetable oil are added to the finished dishes.

6.5.8.1.6 Excluded foods

- Fatty meats and fish.
- The internal organs of animals.
- Refractory fats (pork, lamb, goose, and duck).
- Fatty fish species (halibut, catfish, sturgeon, etc.).
- Confectionery with cream, muffin, brown bread, and millet.
- Coffee: cocoa, chocolate, and ice cream.
- Spices: spices, pickles, marinades.
- Sour varieties of fruits and berries, raw vegetables and fruits.
- Legumes, rutabaga, sorrel, spinach, mushrooms, white cabbage, vegetables rich in essential oils (onions, garlic, radish, radish), nuts, and seeds.
- Broths, egg yolks, canned meat, and fish.
- Alcohol.
- Carbonated drinks.

6.5.8.1.7 Diet N°5a in the Presence of ascites

In ascites, it is recommended to prescribe a diet with a reduced energy value of up to 1500–2000 kcal, containing 70 g of protein and not more than 22 mmol of sodium per day (0.5 g). Diet should be essentially vegetarian. Most high protein foods also contain a lot of sodium. The diet needs to be supplemented with low sodium protein foods. Eat salt-free bread and butter. All dishes are prepared without adding salt.

6.5.8.1.8 Approximate One-Day Diet Menu for a Patient with Ascites

Energy value 2000–2200kcal, protein content up to 70g, sodium content 18–20mmol (380–450mg) per day. The amount of free fluid should not exceed 1 liter.

- Breakfast. Semolina porridge with cream and sugar or baked fruit/60g of saltless bread, or bread, or saltless crackers with unsalted butter and marmalade (jelly or honey). 1 egg, tea or coffee with milk.

- Dinner. 60g of beef or poultry meat or 90g of white fish. Potatoes. Greens or lettuce. Fruits (fresh or baked).

- An afternoon snack. 60g of salt-free bread or bread. Unsalted butter, jam, honey or tomato. Tea or coffee with milk.

- Dinner. Soup without salt or grapefruit. Beef, poultry, fish (as for lunch). Potatoes, greens or leaf lettuce fruits (fresh or baked) or jelly made from fruit juice and gelatin. Sour cream. Tea or coffee with milk.

6.5.8.2 Diet N°5b

6.5.8.2.1 Indications

With prolonged exacerbations of cholecystitis, especially with severe pain resulting from an acute inflammatory process in the gall bladder and surrounding tissues, an anti-inflammatory diet N°5c is recommended.

6.5.8.2.2 General Characteristics

In diet N°5c, carbohydrates are sharply limited to 200g (instead of 400-500g in diet N°5), especially due to easily absorbed (sugar, honey, jam), the protein content is reduced to 80g, the amount of fat is up to 40g. Food is prepared without adding salt, it is given only mashed in the form of soufflé, mashed potatoes, and mucous soups. It is very important to provide a large amount of vitamin C in the daily diet, which is achieved by the inclusion of a rosehip broth.

Diet N°5c is recommended for a short period (4-5 days), usually for the period until the patient is forced to observe strict bed rest, then the patient is transferred to diet N°5a for 1-2 weeks, and then to diet N°5.

6.5.8.2.3 Approximate One-Day Diet Menu

- First breakfast. Protein omelet - 100g. Baked apple - 100g. Tea with milk - 1 cup.

- Lunch. Baked apple - 100g. Carrot juice - ½ cup.

- Dinner. Mucous soup - half a plate. Souffle meat, steam - 125g. Fruit jelly - 125g.

- An afternoon snack. Rosehip broth - 1 cup. White crackers with sugar.

- Dinner. Steam fish souffle - 125g. Baked apple - 100g. Tea with milk - 1 cup.

- Before bedtime. Baked apple. Rosehip broth - 1 cup.

- All-day. Dried wheat bread - 200g, sugar - 40g.

6.5.8.3 Diet N°5c

Two options of a diet N°5c are used.

6.5.8.3.1 First version

It is used for acute pancreatitis and chronic pancreatitis in the stage of sharp exacerbation.

The purpose of this diet is creating maximum functional rest of the pancreas and relieving pain. Mechanical sparing of the stomach, duodenum, and intestines, a decrease in the reflex excitability of the gall bladder.

The diet, mechanically and biochemically as sparing as possible, is prescribed after hungry days. In view of the insufficient content of the main nutrients in comparison with physiological norms and the needs of the body, this variant of the pancreatic diet is usually prescribed for 3-7 days.

Frequent (6–8 times/day) meals are recommended in small portions (not more than 300g).

Food should be steamed or boiled, and have a semi-liquid consistency. The diet should be complete with vitamin and mineral composition.

The temperature of the prepared dishes is 20–52 °C.

6.5.8.3.1.1 Composition

Proteins 60-80g (of which 25g of animal protein), fats 50-60g, carbohydrates 200-280g; calorie content of 1490-1780kcal; retinol 0.3mg, carotene 10mg, thiamine 1.3mg, riboflavin 2mg, nicotinic acid 1-6mg, ascorbic acid 150mg; sodium 3g, calcium 0.8g, magnesium 0.5g, phosphorus 1.3g, iron 0.030g. This table has a relatively low-calorie content (up to 1800kcal) due to the sharp restriction of animal proteins, fats, and carbohydrates. The daily intake of table salt is 6-10g, free fluid - up to 2 liters.

6.5.8.3.1.2 Recommended foods

Prescribe mainly carbohydrate nutrition in the form of mashed cereals on water, mucous soups from various cereals, tea with sugar, crackers (up to 50g/day), jelly or mousse from juice on xylitol, vegetable puree (potato, carrot, pumpkin, squash) without adding oil or steam vegetable puddings, and semi-liquid mashed jelly from fruit. Bread is allowed white, yesterday, dry cookies.

After the removal of acute phenomena and the reduction of pain, the diet gradually expands and is prescribed in the form of the second option.

6.5.8.3.1.3 Excluded foods

All foods and dishes not listed above are excluded from the diet of patients. From the daily diet, it is necessary to exclude all products that cause bloating, roughage, as well as products that enhance the secretion of digestive juices.

6.5.8.3.2 The Second version

It is prescribed for acute pancreatitis in the phase of subsiding of the main manifestations of the disease and chronic pancreatitis in the phase of mild exacerbation.

When the exacerbation of pancreatitis subsides, it is important to prevent the development of relapse and progression of pancreatitis, as well as to correct the nutritional disorders that have arisen.

This diet contains a high protein content, a reduced amount of fat and simple carbohydrates, a restriction of extractive substances and crude fiber. Fractional (5–6 times/day) nutrition is kept in small portions. The diet is prescribed for 2-3 months, gradually increasing the amount of food and the list of products and dishes. All dishes are boiled or steamed, and crushed.

With deterioration in well-being, the patient return to the first version of this diet.

6.5.8.3.2.1 Composition

Protein 110-120g. On average, the protein content in the diet is 1.4-1.5g/kg of normal body weight. With pronounced weight loss, the daily protein quota is increased to 130g. Fat 70g (the fat content in the diet is at the lower boundary of the physiological norm), 20% are vegetable fats, carbohydrates 350-400g (simple carbohydrates limit to 30g), calorie content 2470-2700kcal; retinol 0.4mg, carotene 12.8mg, thiamine 1.4mg, riboflavin 2.6mg, nicotinic acid 17mg, ascorbic acid 250mg; sodium 4g, potassium 4.0g, calcium 1.3g, magnesium 0.48g, phosphorus 1.9g, iron 0.035g. The amount of sodium chloride is limited to 6–8g/day. The amount of permissible free fluid remains the same - 1.5–2l/day.

6.5.8.3.2.2 Recommended foods

- Wheat bread from yesterday's flour I and II or dried.

- Meat and poultry - low-fat varieties of beef, veal, rabbit; chicken, boiled turkey, mashed and chopped.

- Fish - low-fat varieties, boiled in a piece or chopped.

- Souffle from meat and river fish of non-fat varieties (beef, veal, chicken, turkey, rabbit, cod, pike perch, carp, perch, pike, etc.), meatballs, dumplings or meatballs.

- With poor tolerance of animal proteins, it is advisable to use soy protein.

- Eggs - in the form of protein steam omelets or soft-boiled egg (no more than 1-2 eggs/day).

- Dairy products - fresh cottage cheese of low-fat content. Some doctors allow the use of milk in the absence of lactase deficiency, but only in dishes. Sour cream and cream in small quantities only in the dish. Steam curd pudding. Calcined cottage cheese is indicated for persons with calcium deficiency.

- Cereals - mashed and semi-viscous cereals made from oat, buckwheat and semolina, rice, cooked on water or in half with milk. Semi-liquid porridge from oatmeal.

- Vegetables - Potatoes, carrots, beets, boiled or baked cauliflower. Soybeans are recommended.

- In order to prevent intestinal dysbiosis, some authors recommend the introduction into the radio 100-200g of raw vegetables (carrots, cabbage, and celery) up to 2-3 times a day.

- Sauces - milk, fruit, and berry.

- Drinks: weak tea with lemon and xylitol, broth of wild rose.

- Patients with potassium deficiency are recommended carrot juice and dried fruit compotes.

- Baked sweet apples are allowed (Antonov and other sour varieties are excluded), fruit drinks and infusions of dried and mashed fresh non-acidic fruits and berries rich in potassium salts.

- Of sweet foods, fruit and berry juices without sugar, diluted with water, stewed fruit with fresh pulp and dried fruit (apples, pears, and apricots), jelly, mousse of juices on xylitol or sorbate, pastille, and jelly marmalade are allowed.

- With good tolerance of the second variant of diet N°5c in the future (after 3-5 days), fats are added to the patient's diet, first in the form of unsalted butter, added to prepared cereals and vegetable purees (up to 15–20g during the day), then refined sunflower oil (up to 5-15g/day).

6.5.8.3.2.3 Excluded foods

- Excluded from the menu are foods rich in extractive substances, oxalic acid, and essential oils that stimulate the secretory activity of the stomach and pancreas.

- Meat, fish and mushroom broths, and salted cabbage soup are excluded.

- Fatty varieties of meat and fish, liver, kidneys, brains, smoked meats, salted fish, caviar, most sausages, and canned foods are undesirable.

- Pork, beef, and lamb; cooking fats are excluded.

- Goose, duck, liver, kidneys, brains, smoked meats, sausages, canned meat, and fish are excluded; fatty varieties of meat, poultry, fish.

- Hard-boiled and fried eggs are excluded.

- Fresh bread is excluded. Puff pastry and pastry, pastries, cakes, and fried pastries remain prohibited.

- Cream, milk 6% fat is excluded.

- Legumes, sorrel, radishes, green onions, garlic, mushrooms, and pickled vegetables are excluded.

- Extreme caution should be taken with hot spices: horseradish, mustard, pepper, and ketchup.

- Excluded also are: chocolate, cream products, black coffee, and cocoa.

- Absolute rejection of alcoholic beverages is necessary.

6.5.8.3.2.4   Sample menu of the second version

At the initial stage

- 1st breakfast: calcined cottage cheese pudding, milk oatmeal porridge, and tea.

- 2nd breakfast: boiled tongue, rosehip broth, and crackers.

- Lunch: milk soup with semolina, steamed meat patties, carrot puree, and compote from mashed dried fruits.

- Snack: fish cutlets with rice and fruit juice jelly.

- Dinner: calcified cottage cheese, meatloaf stuffed with scrambled eggs, steam, and tea with milk.

- At night: kefir.

- For the whole day: yesterday's wheat bread baking - 200g, sugar - 20g.

Advanced stage

- 1st breakfast: protein omelet, milk buckwheat porridge, cheese, and tea.

- 2nd breakfast: boiled meat souffle, rosehip broth, and crackers.

- Lunch: meatball soup, stewed chicken with boiled rice, a salad of fresh cucumbers and tomatoes, and fruit compote.

- Snack: cottage cheese and rice casserole, peach juice.

- Dinner: a salad of grated carrots, boiled cod with white sauce, mashed potatoes, and tea.

- At night: kefir.

- For the whole day: 100g rye bread, 200g wheat bread, 20g butter, and 40g sugar.

6.5.8.4 Diet N°5d

Prescribed mainly for post-cholecystectomy syndrome in the acute stage, accompanied by concomitant duodenitis, exacerbation of chronic gastritis, and hepatitis.

6.5.8.4.1 Purpose

Maximum sparing of the liver and other digestive organs, a decrease in the intensity of bile secretion.

6.5.8.4.2 General characteristics

A diet with a reduced-calorie content, a normal content of easily digestible proteins and a significant restriction of fats, with the exception of vegetable oil, foods containing large amounts of cholesterol; with the restriction of easily absorbed carbohydrates and the exclusion of nitrogenous extractives, purines, and coarse fiber.

Fractional (5-6 times/day) food in small portions.

The diet is designed to reduce body weight, which in these patients is often overweight, and improve lipid metabolism. All dishes are boiled or steam mashed; frying is excluded. Once a week, a fasting day is possible.

6.5.8.4.3 Composition

Protein 90g, fat 60g (vegetable fat excluded), carbohydrates 300g (simple carbohydrates limit to 30-50g); calories 2000-2200kcal; retinol 0.3mg, carotene 6.7mg, thiamine 1mg, riboflavin 1.5mg, nicotinic acid 13mg, ascorbic acid 100mg; sodium 3.5g, potassium 3g, calcium 0.35g, phosphorus 1.2g, iron 0.04g. The amount of sodium chloride is limited to 6g (of which 3g is in products). The amount of permissible free fluid remains the same - 1.5–2l/day.

6.5.8.4.4 Recommended foods

- Yesterday's wheat bread and crackers from wheat bread.

- Snacks - mild cheese.

- Soups mashed from vegetables, cereals on a vegetable broth; mashed soup of carrots, cauliflower.

- Meat and fish - low-fat varieties of meat, fish in the form of soufflé, dumplings, steam cutlets; a chicken from cookware is allowed a piece.

- Eggs - 1 egg per day - protein steam omelet, protein souffle.

- Milk and dairy products: milk with good tolerance, low-fat fresh cottage cheese in the form of soufflé, puddings, and sour cream only as a seasoning.

- Vegetables - potatoes, pumpkin, cauliflower, zucchini, boiled, baked and stewed carrots.

- Fruits and berries are ripe, sweet varieties in the form of mashed compotes, jelly, and mousse.

- Sweets - sharply limited.

- Sauces are dairy, sour cream, and fruit sauce.

- Drinks - fruit, berry juices, and decoctions.

6.5.8.4.5 Excluded foods

Fatty meat and fish, raw vegetables and fruits, radishes, onions, garlic, meat, fish and mushroom broths are prohibited.

6.5.8.5 Diet N°5e

This diet is efficient in chronic liver disease, accompanied by a stagnation of bile, a condition after cholecystectomy with the presence of cholesterol syndrome and hypomotor biliary dyskinesia.

6.5.8.5.1 Purpose

Strengthening bile secretion, improving the hepatic and intestinal circulation of bile components, providing lipotropic effects, introducing high-grade proteins and polyunsaturated fatty acids into the diet.

6.5.8.5.2 General characteristics

A physiologically complete diet with a normal protein, carbohydrate content (simple carbohydrates limit) and a high-fat diet, enriched with lipotropic factors.

Food is cooked in water, steamed or baked. Food chopping is optional. Roasting is excluded. Fractional (5-6 times/day) food in small portions.

6.5.8.5.3 Composition

Proteins 100g, fats 110-120g (50% vegetable fat), carbohydrates 350-400g; calorie content 2800-3160kcal; retinol 0.3mg, carotene 10.3mg, thiamine 1.7mg, riboflavin 2.5mg, nicotinic acid 18.5mg, ascorbic acid 200mg; sodium 3.7g, potassium 4.45g, calcium 1.3g, magnesium 0.55g, phosphorus 1.6g, and iron 0.040g. Consumption of sodium chloride should be limited to 8g per day. The amount of permissible free fluid remains the same - 1.5–2l/day.

6.5.8.5.4 Recommended foods

- Yesterday's wheat, rye bread, and bran bread.
- Fats - butter, ghee, olive, and corn. The ratio of animal to vegetable fat is 1:1.
- Snacks are mild and unsalted.
- Soups - vegetarian, cereals, dairy, borscht, and beetroot soup.
- Meat dishes from low-fat varieties of beef, chicken, turkey in the form of beef stroganoff from boiled meat; meatballs, dumplings, and chicken meatballs steamed or baked.
- Fish - dishes from low-fat varieties in boiled and baked form, in the form of soufflé, knives, and cutlets - steam and baked.
- Eggs and dishes from them - soft-boiled egg or scrambled eggs.
- Dishes from cereals and pasta - crumbly and viscous cereals from semolina, rice, buckwheat, and oatmeal.
- Boiled and baked vegetables.

- Fruits and berries are ripe, sweet in raw form.
- Sweets - sugar, jam, and honey.

6.5.8.5.5 Excluded foods

Meat and fish of fatty varieties, spicy vegetables, internal organs of animals, garlic, onions, chocolate, cocoa, carbonated, and alcoholic drinks.

6.5.8.6 Diet N°5f

6.5.8.6.1 Indications

Surgery on the stomach. Dumping syndrome after resection of the stomach for peptic ulcer.

6.5.8.6.2 General characteristics

A physiologically complete diet with an increased amount of protein, amount of fat, a restriction of complex carbohydrates to the lower limit of the norm, and complete exclusion of easily absorbed carbohydrates. In the diet, the consumption of chemical stimulants of gastric and pancreatic secretion, irritants of the mucous membrane and receptors of the gastrointestinal tract is limited. All dishes are cooked boiled or steamed. Food is given in a warm form, very hot and cold dishes are excluded. The dietary intake should be fractionated to 6–7 times a day. If possible, go to bed 15-30 minutes after eating, especially after lunch.

With severe dumping syndrome, the effect of eating food in a horizontal position of the patient, better on the left side.

With positive dynamics, the non-rubbed version of the diet is expanded: it is allowed to increase the consumption of table salt up to 10-15g per day, chemical stimulants are introduced into the diet. Fried foods are allowed, but without a rough crust.

Fluids should be taken separately from other dishes, i.e. tea, milk, the third dish at lunch and kefir in the evening should be consumed 20-30 minutes after the main meal. The amount of fluid at one time should not be plentiful (no more than 1 glass).

The options for diet N°5f have been developed: the rubbed version, the non-rubbed version, and the intermediate version. All options have the same composition; only the technological processing of food changes. When wiped, all dishes are wiped after steaming. In the intermediate version: fish, meat is given in chopped form, and the side dishes are in an unpasted form, with a viscous consistency (mashed gruel, mashed potatoes). Salads, fresh fruits, and vegetables are excluded, only stale white bread and white crackers are also provided. In the non-mashed version, the diet expands, non-mashed meat and fish dishes, non-mashed soups, salads, fruits, and vegetables are introduced.

6.5.8.6.3 Composition

Protein 120g, 90g fat, 400g carbohydrates, total calorie content - 2850kcal. Consumption of salt should be limited to 8g per day.

6.5.8.6.4 Recommended foods

- Bread and bread products - yesterday's white wheat bread, white crackers, low-acid buns, and non-butter biscuits.

- Snacks - cheese is spicy, grated, ham - scalloped, low-fat.

- Soups - mashed from cereals, mashed soup of vegetables on a weak vegetable broth, soup with noodles - 1-2 plates.

- Meat and fish dishes - from beef (low-fat), veal, chicken, pike perch, carp, perch and other low-fat fish varieties in boiled and steam form. Beef is minced or cooked in the Ostroganov style.

- Dishes from eggs - soft-boiled egg, steam omelet, not more than 1 egg per day.

- Milk and dairy products - fresh, dried, condensed milk without sugar is added to dishes; in minimal quantities, fresh, non-acidic sour cream; fresh non-acidic mashed cottage cheese (with intolerance completely excluded).

- Dishes and side dishes of cereals and pasta - unsweetened, mashed cereals, milk (1/3 milk), unsweetened puddings, steamed, boiled vermicelli, finely chopped pasta, and boiled, home-cooked noodles (limited).

- Dishes and side dishes from vegetables and leafy greens - vegetable puree (except cabbage), vegetable steam puddings, zucchini and pumpkin, boiled vegetables with butter.

- Sweet dishes and pastries - sugar, honey, and jam are limited.

- Fruits and berries are unsweetened varieties of ripe fruits and berries in the form of mashed unsweetened compotes, jelly, and mousses.

- Fats - butter, melted unsalted, olive oil.

- Juices are given in the form of raw non-acidic and unsweetened fruit, berry, vegetable juices, and a decoction of rose hips. Grape juice is limited.

6.5.8.6.5 Excluded foods

- Eliminate difficult to tolerate fatty foods: goose meat, duck, fatty pork, lamb, and various types of lard.

- Exclude meat, fish and strong vegetable decoctions, especially mushroom.

- Don't allow liver, brains, kidneys, lungs, pickles, smoked meats, marinades, all kinds of spicy snacks, sausages, canned meat, and fish snacks.

- Exclude pastry, pies, and brown bread.

- Raw uncooked vegetables and fruits are excluded.

- Ice cream, chocolate, cocoa, any alcoholic drinks are not allowed.

- Restriction of foods and dishes that most often cause dumping syndrome: sweets (sugar, honey, jam), very hot or very cold dishes, liquid sweet milk porridges, etc.

6.5.8.6.6 One-day diet menu for a patient with severe dumping syndrome (in the long-term period of the post-stationary rehabilitation phase)

- 1st breakfast: boiled meat, sauerkraut salad in vegetable oil, half a cup of tea without sugar.
- 2nd breakfast: loose buckwheat porridge.
- 3rd breakfast: meat steams and fresh apple.
- Lunch: vegetarian cabbage soup 1/2 plates (200g) and boiled meat.
- Snack: protein omelet and jelly on xylitol.
- Dinner: fresh cottage cheese (100g), kefir (1 cup).
- At night: kefir, calcified curd.
- For the whole day: rye bread 100g, white bread 100g.

6.5.8.6.2 One-day diet menu

- 1st breakfast: steam protein omelet, buckwheat cereal without sugar, and tea.
- 2nd breakfast: steamed meat patties and baked apple without sugar.

- Lunch: vegetarian oat soup, boiled chicken with mashed potatoes, and fruit jelly without sugar.

- Snack: boiled fish.

- Dinner: meat steamroll, stewed carrots, and cottage cheese pudding without sugar.

- At night: kefir, calcified curd.

- For the whole day: white bread - 300g, white crackers - 50g.

6.5.8.6.3 One-day diet of the non-rubbed diet without biochemical sparing

- 1st breakfast: fried meatballs, fresh cabbage salad in vegetable oil, loose buckwheat porridge, and tea with milk.

- 2nd breakfast: cheese 50g and fresh apple.

- Lunch: cabbage soup on meat broth, stew with boiled potatoes, and jelly on xylitol.

- Snack: 2 egg omelets and rosehip broth.

- Dinner: boiled fish with stewed carrots and cheesecake with cottage cheese without sugar.

- At night: kefir 1 cup and fresh curd 100g.

- For the whole day: rye bread 150-200g, white bread 150g, sugar 40g.

AUTHOR'S PRESENTATION

Dr. Amin Gasmi is a physiologist and orthomolecular nutritionist. He is currently the president of the Francophone Society of Nutritherapy and Applied Nutrigenetics. He is also the founder and managing editor of the International Journal of Integrative Physiology and Nutritional Sciences. He is a member of several international scientific organizations such as the International Society of Immunonutrition and the International Society of Orthomolecular Medicine. Dr. Gasmi has a multidisciplinary background and had the opportunity to work on several fields such as nutrition sciences, micronutrition, genetics, exercise physiology, applied psychology, physical therapy, physical training, and biochemistry. He has a triple competence of clinician through patients' and athletes' nutritional and physiological care, of scientist through his high quality published books and articles, and of professional trainer through the trainings and lectures he gives to medical doctors, health, and sports professionals.

REFERENCES

Alverdy J. (1994). The effect of nutrition on gastrointestinal barrier function. Semin Respir Infect. 9(4):248-55.

Barnes J. L. (2018). Enteral Nutrients and Gastrointestinal Physiology. J. Infus Nurs. 41(1):35-42.

Bielawska B., Allard J. P. (2017). Parenteral Nutrition and Intestinal Failure. Nutrients. 9(5):466.

Chandler M. (2013). Focus on nutrition: dietary management of gastrointestinal disease. Compend Contin Educ Vet. 35(6): E1-3.

Eswaran S., Farida S., Green J., Miller J. D., Chey W. D. (2017). Nutrition in the management of gastrointestinal diseases and disorders: the evidence for the low FODMAP diet. Curr Opin Pharmacol. 37:151-157.

Gilliland T. M., Villafane-Ferriol N., Shah K. P., Shah R. M., Tran Cao H. S., Massarweh N. N., Silberfein E. J., Choi E. A., Hsu C., McElhany A. L., Barakat O., Fisher W., Van Buren G. (2017). Nutritional and Metabolic Derangements in Pancreatic Cancer and Pancreatic Resection. Nutrients. 9(3):243.

Hasse J. M. (2008). Nutrition in clinical practice. Gastrointestinal disorders and their connections to nutrition. Nutr Clin Pract. 23(3):259.

Jankowski M., Las-Jankowska M., Sousak M., Zegarski W. (2018). Contemporary enteral and parenteral nutrition before surgery for gastrointestinal cancers: a literature review. World J. Surg Oncol. 16(1):94.

Jeejeebhoy K. N. (1998). Nutritional assessment. Gastroenterol Clin North Am. 27(2):347-69.

Le Gall M., Thenet S., Aguanno D., Jarry A. C., Genser L., Ribeiro-Parenti L., Joly F., Ledoux S., Bado A., - Le Beyec J. (2019). Intestinal plasticity in response to nutrition and gastrointestinal surgery. Nutr Rev. 77(3):129-143.

Mandato C., Di Nuzzi A., Vajro P (2017). Nutrition and Liver Disease. Nutrients. 10(1):9.

Merli M., Berzigotti A., Zelber-Sagi S., Dasarathy S., Montagnese S., Genton L., Plauth M., Pares A. (2019). EASL Clinical Practice Guidelines on nutrition in chronic liver disease. J Hepatol. 70(1):172-193.

Morgenroth K., Kozuschek W., Holtz J. (1991). Pancreatitis, Walter de Gruyter, Berlin-New York

Pan L. L., Li J., Shamoon M., Bhatia M., Sun J. (2017). Recent Advances on Nutrition in Treatment of Acute Pancreatitis. Front Immunol. 8:762.

Rasmussen H. H., Irtun O., Olesen S. S., Drewes A. M., Holst M. (2013). Nutrition in chronic pancreatitis. World J. Gastroenterol. 19(42):7267–7275.

Schörghuber M., Fruhwald S. (2018). Effects of enteral nutrition on gastrointestinal function in patients who are critically ill. Lancet Gastroenterol Hepatol. 3(4):281-287.

Shergill R., Syed W., Rizvi S. A., Singh I (2018). Nutritional support in chronic liver disease and cirrhotics. World J Hepatol. 10(10):685–694.

Shu X. L., Kang K., Gu L. J., Zhang Y. S. (2016). Effect of early enteral nutrition on patients with digestive tract surgery: A meta-analysis of randomized controlled trials. Exp Ther Med. 12(4):2136–2144.

Silva M., Gomes S., Peixoto A., Torres-Ramalho P., Cardoso H., Azevedo R., Cunha C., Macedo G. (2015). Nutrition in Chronic Liver Disease. GE Port J Gastroenterol. 22(6):268-276.

Storck L. J., Imoberdorf R., Ballmer P. E. (2019). Nutrition in Gastrointestinal Disease: Liver, Pancreatic, and Inflammatory Bowel Disease. J Clin Med. 25;8(8).

Tomasello G., Mazzola M., Leone A., Sinagra E., Zummo G., Farina F., Damiani P., Cappello F., Gerges Geagea A., Jurjus A., Bou Assi T., Messina M., Carini F. (2016). Nutrition, oxidative stress and intestinal dysbiosis: Influence of diet on gut microbiota in inflammatory bowel diseases. Biomed Pap Med Fac Univ Palacky Olomouc Czech Repub. 160(4):461-466.

Walters J. R. F. (2007). Clinical nutrition in gastrointestinal disease. Gut. 56(10): 1487–1488.

www.ingramcontent.com/pod-product-compliance
Lightning Source LLC
Chambersburg PA
CBHW052347220526
45465CB00003BA/1001